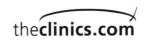
the**clinics**.com

SURGICAL CLINICS
OF NORTH AMERICA

Evidence-Based Surgery

GUEST EDITORS
Jonathan L. Meakins, OC, MD, DSc,
FRCS(Hon), FRCS(C,Glas)
Sir Muir Gray, CBE, DSc, MD, FRCP,
FRCPS(Glas)

CONSULTING EDITOR
Ronald F. Martin, MD

February 2006 • Volume 86 • Number 1

SAUNDERS

An Imprint of Elsevier, Inc.
PHILADELPHIA   LONDON   TORONTO   MONTREAL   SYDNEY   TOKYO

W.B. SAUNDERS COMPANY
A Division of Elsevier Inc.

1600 John F. Kennedy Blvd., Suite 1800, Philadelphia, PA 19103-2899

http://www.theclinics.com

SURGICAL CLINICS OF NORTH AMERICA   Volume 86, Number 1
February 2006   ISSN 0039–6109
Editor: Catherine Bewick   ISBN 1-4160-3557-5

The ideas and opinions expressed in *The Surgical Clinics of North America* do not necessarily reflect those of the Publisher. The Publisher does not assume any responsibility for any injury and/or damage to persons or property arising out of or related to any use of the material contained in this periodical. The reader is advised to check the appropriate medical literature and the product information currently provided by the manufacturer of each drug to be administered to verify the dosage, the method and duration of administration, or contraindications. It is the responsibility of the treating physician or other health care professional, relying on independent experience and knowledge of the patient, to determine drug dosages and the best treatment for the patient. Mention of any product in this issue should not be construed as endorsement by the contributors, editors, or the Publisher of the product or manufacturers' claims.

Surgical Clinics of North America (ISSN 0039–6109) is published bimonthly by Elsevier; Corporate and editorial Offices: 1600 John F. Kennedy Blvd., Suite 1800, Philadelphia, PA 19103-2899. Accounting and circulation offices: 6277 Sea Harbor Drive, Orlando, FL 32887-4800. Periodicals postage paid at Orlando, FL 32862, and additional mailing offices. Subscription prices are $200.00 per year for US individuals, $315.00 per year for US institutions, $100.00 per year for US students and residents, $245.00 per year for Canadian individuals, $385.00 per year for Canadian institutions, $260.00 for international individuals, $385.00 for international institutions and $130.00 per year for Canadian and foreign students/residents. To receive student/resident rate, orders must be accompanied by name of affiliated institution, date of term, and the *signature* of program/residency coordinator on institution letterhead. Orders will be billed at individual rate until proof of status is received. Foreign air speed delivery is included in all *Clinics* subscription prices. All prices are subject to change without notice. POSTMASTER: Send address changes to *The Surgical Clinics of North America*, W.B. Saunders Company, Periodicals Fulfillment, Orlando, FL 32887-4800. **Customer Service: 1-800-654-2452 (US). From outside of the US, call 1-407-345-1000.**

The Surgical Clinics of North America is also published in Spanish by McGraw-Hill Interamericana Editores S.A., P.O. Box 5-237 06500 Mexico D.F. Mexico; and in Portuguese by Interlivros Edicoes Ltda., Rua Comandante Coelho 1085, CEP 21250, Rio de Janeiro, Brazil; and in Greek by Paschalidis Medical Publications, Athens Greece.

The Surgical Clinics of North America is covered in *Index Medicus, EMBASE/Excerpta Medica, Current Contents/Clinical Medicine, Current Contents/Life Sciences, Science Citation Index,* and *ISI/BIOMED.*

Printed in the United States of America.

CONSULTING EDITOR

RONALD F. MARTIN, MD, Staff Surgeon, Department of Surgery, Marshfield Clinic, Marshfield, Wisconsin; Clinical Associate Professor of Surgery, University of Vermont, Burlington, Vermont; Lieutenant Colonel, Medical Corps, United States Army Reserve

GUEST EDITORS

JONATHAN L. MEAKINS, OC, MD, DSc, FRCS(Hon), FRCS(C,Glas), Nuffield Professor of Surgery, Nuffield Department of Surgery, John Radcliffe Hospital, University of Oxford, Oxford, England, United Kingdom

SIR MUIR GRAY, CBE, DSc, MD, FRCP, FRCPS(Glas), Nuffield Department of Surgery, University of Oxford, Oxford, England, United Kingdom

CONTRIBUTORS

WENDY J. BABIDGE, BAppSci(Hons), PhD, Program Manager, Australian Safety and Efficacy Register of New Interventional Procedures–Surgical (ASERNIP-S), Royal Australasian College of Surgeons; Department of Surgery, University of Adelaide, The Queen Elizabeth Hospital, Adelaide, South Australia, Australia

DOUGLAS BADENOCH, MSc, Director, Minervation Ltd, Oxford, England, United Kingdom

JEFFREY S. BARKUN, MD, MSc, Department of Surgery, McGill University; Royal Victoria Hospital, Montreal, Quebec, Canada

SIMON BERGMAN, MD, MSc, Department of Surgery, McGill University; Montreal General Hospital, Montreal, Quebec, Canada

ANNE BRICE, BA(Hons), Dip. Lib., MCLIP, Acting Head of Service, National Library for Health, University of Oxford, Headington, Oxford, England, United Kingdom

INGRID BURGER, BS, Department of Health Policy and Management, Johns Hopkins Bloomberg School of Public Health, Baltimore, Maryland

MARTIN BURTON MA, DM, FRCS, Consultant Otolaryngologist, Senior Clinical Lecturer, University of Oxford; Coordinating Editor, Cochrane Ear, Nose and Throat Disorders Group; Department of Otolaryngology-Head and Neck Surgery, the Radcliffe Infirmary, Oxford, England, United Kingdom

MIKE CLARKE, MA, DPhil, Director, United Kingdom Cochrane Centre, Oxford, England, United Kingdom

LIANE S. FELDMAN, MD, Department of Surgery, McGill University; Montreal General Hospital, Montreal, Quebec, Canada

PAUL GLASZIOU, MD, PhD, Director, Centre for Evidence-Based Practice, Department of Primary Health Care; University of Oxford, Oxford, England, United Kingdom

STEVEN N. GOODMAN, MD, PhD, Associate Professor, Phoebe Berman Bioethics Institute, The Johns Hopkins University; Departments of Epidemiology and Biostatistics, Johns Hopkins Bloomberg School of Public Health; Department of Oncology, The Johns Hopkins University School of Medicine, Baltimore, Maryland

SIR MUIR GRAY, CBE, DSc, MD, FRCP, FRCPS(Glas), Nuffield Department of Surgery, University of Oxford, Oxford, England, United Kingdom

R. SCOTT JONES, MD, FACS, Professor, Department of Surgery, University of Virginia Health System, Charlottesville, Virginia; Director, Division of Research and Optimal Patient Care, American College of Surgeons, Chicago, Illinois

THALIA KNIGHT, MA (Rhodes), MA (London), MCLIP, Head of Library and Information Services, The Royal College of Surgeons of England, London, England, United Kingdom

MARTIN J.R. LEE, MA, MSc, FRCS, Medical Director and Consultant Surgeon, University Hospitals, Coventry and Warwickshire National Health Service Trust, Walsgrave Hospital, Coventry, England, United Kingdom

GUY J. MADDERN, PhD, MD, FRACS, Surgical Director, Australian Safety and Efficacy Register of New Interventional Procedures–Surgical (ASERNIP-S), Royal Australasian College of Surgeons; RP Jepson Professor of Surgery, Department of Surgery, University of Adelaide, Queen Elizabeth Hospital, Adelaide, South Australia, Australia

JOHN C. MARSHALL, MD, FRCSC, Professor of Surgery, Departments of Surgery and Critical Care Medicine, University of Toronto, Toronto, Ontario, Canada

PETER McCULLOCH, MD, FRCSEd, Clinical Reader in Surgery, Nuffield Department of Surgery, John Radcliffe Hospital, Oxford University, Oxford, England, United Kingdom

JONATHAN L. MEAKINS, OC, MD, DSc, FRCS(Hon), FRCS(C,Glas), Nuffield Professor of Surgery, Nuffield Department of Surgery, John Radcliffe Hospital, University of Oxford, Oxford, England, United Kingdom

PHILLIPA F. MIDDLETON, BSc(Hons), GradDipLibStud, MPH, Research Manager, Australian Safety and Efficacy Register of New Interventional Procedures–Surgical (ASERNIP-S), Royal Australasian College of Surgeons, Adelaide, South Australia, Australia

ALBERT G. MULLEY, JR, MD, Chief, General Medicine Division; Director, Medical Practice Evaluation Center, Massachusetts General Hospital; Associate Professor of Medicine; Associate Professor of Health Policy, Harvard Medical School, Boston, Massachusetts

KAREN RICHARDS, BA, Administrative Director, Division of Research and Optimal Patient Care, American College of Surgeons, Chicago, Illinois

THOMAS RUSSELL, MD, FACS, Executive Director, American College of Surgeons, Chicago, Illinois

NICK SEVDALIS, BSc, MSc, PhD, Research Associate, Division of Surgery, Imperial College, St. Mary's Campus, London, England, United Kingdom

JEREMY SUGARMAN, MD, MPH, MA, Professor, Department of Health Policy and Management, Johns Hopkins Bloomberg School of Public Health; Phoebe Berman Bioethics Institute, The Johns Hopkins University; Department of Medicine, The Johns Hopkins University School of Medicine, Baltimore, Maryland

REBECCA TOOHER, BA, PGDipAud, PhD, Senior Research Officer, Australian Safety and Efficacy Register of New Interventional Procedures–Surgical (ASERNIP-S), Royal Australasian College of Surgeons, Adelaide, South Australia, Australia

CONTENTS

> Understanding the issues associated with surgical epidemiology, knowledge management, and evidence-based surgical practice has implications for clinicians in the community, surgeons in large metropolitan hospitals, surgeon scholars, and the academic surgeon. All need to have some understanding of not only the evaluation of the evidence and how to find it but, in addition, application of those concepts to continuous quality improvement and to closing a circle of surgical audit. If the surgical profession has an obligation to redefine clinical modus operandi and educational processes, the argument for formal training in aspects of clinical epidemiology during the surgical residency program is obvious, because all surgeons will benefit from those educational exercises.

> The yawning gap between what we know and what we do has major implications for patients. By putting into practice what we know now, we will have a bigger impact on the health of individuals and populations than any drug or technology discovered in the new decade. The assumption underlying this article is that the gap can be closed by thinking, planning, analyzing, mobilizing, managing, personalizing, and using knowledge. There is, however,

a risk that the attempted solution may perpetuate or aggravate the problem, and surgeons must be aware of the dangers of substituting thought for action, when knowledge management becomes an industry of its own, remote from the core activities of the organization and those who deliver them.

Developing Skills for Evidence-Based Surgery

Finding and Appraising Evidence 41
Peter McCulloch and Douglas Badenoch

Surgeons have tended to regard evidence-based medicine with a degree of skepticism. A variety of reasons for this have been proposed, ranging from the surgical personality to the nature of the research questions that occur when studying surgical treatment. The relative paucity of randomized trials of surgical treatment has been noted by many investigators, and there has been considerable debate about whether this reflects poorly on the scientific education of the surgical community or points to special problems in applying this methodology in this discipline. This debate has matured over the last 10 years, and there is now greater understanding of the factors that make surgical operations difficult subjects for randomized trials; on the other hand, such trials are being done now more than ever before.

Teaching Evidence-Based Decision-Making 59
Nick Sevdalis and Peter McCulloch

Evidence-based decision-making is important in surgery, but the nature of the work makes it difficult. Teaching it requires an interactive approach with a clinical team willing to consider it seriously, and to derive practical solutions. Decision-making and its influences must be understood, so that surgeons have a realistic idea of the role of evidence. Cognitive factors are particularly important. Strategies developed in the context of this knowledge are more likely to be adopted and used. Experts must be involved in searching for evidence and members of the management team in the learning process, the former to provide expertise on searching, the latter to ensure that the reasons for proposed changes are understood and treated sympathetically by those with financial control.

The Nature of Surgical Evidence

Librarians, Surgeons, and Knowledge 71
Thalia Knight and Anne Brice

This article outlines the increasingly diverse roles undertaken by information professionals in support of the surgical team's knowledge needs for evidence-based practice. Such information professionals may be called "clinical informationists," "information scientists," "information specialists," or "librarians." The role titles are indicative of the ferment of change brought about by the digital revolution, and of the continuing determination of health information professionals to rise to the challenges involved in supporting surgeons and everyone in the surgical team, as they endeavor to provide the best possible care for their patients. Libraries as we know them have changed, and are changing. The scholarly communications process is also undergoing profound transformation. The authors discuss these changes and their implications for surgeons.

Evidence-Based Surgery: Creating the Culture 91
Martin J.R. Lee

Hospitals and professional bodies require a culture that supports surgeons in their quest for knowledge, and provides the technological and educational environment in which they can promote evidence-based surgery. Surgeons must influence the development of their local information technology systems for data collection and outcome analysis, and deliver training programs that instill an attitude of continually seeking evidence. Identification of clinical problems and critical appraisal of the literature need to be taught. Management structures and relationships that facilitate a joint approach to delivering high-quality systematic clinical care should be developed. The culture that supports these aims is also one in which patients can rely on safely receiving up-to-date and effective treatments from well-trained and trusted surgeons.

Producing the Evidence

Systematic Reviews of Surgical Interventions 101
Martin Burton and Mike Clarke

All physicians are familiar with the type of general review articles found in many medical journals. Systematic reviews are different. They apply a strict, scientific methodology to the reviewing process to produce a review that is comprehensive, reliable, and as free from bias as possible. As a result, systematic reviews occupy the highest position in the "levels of evidence" tables associated with the practice of evidence-based health care. Systematic reviews relevant to surgery are no less relevant than systematic reviews in other areas of health care. They should be a prerequisite of any new research, a key component in decision making, and an opportunity for all surgical practitioners to get involved in the conduct and interpretation of research.

Evaluating New Surgical Techniques in Australia: The Australian Safety and Efficacy Register of New Interventional Procedures–Surgical Experience 115
Guy J. Maddern, Philippa F. Middleton, Rebecca Tooher, and Wendy J. Babidge

The Australian Safety and Efficacy Register of New Interventional Procedures–Surgical (ASERNIP–S) exists primarily to assess new surgical technologies and techniques. It originally conducted systematic literature reviews, but now uses accelerated reviews, horizon scanning for emerging procedures, research and clinical audits, preparation of patient information, assistance with guideline development, and the production of research protocols of new surgical techniques. Future international cooperation and networking among health technology assessment groups will avoid duplication of effort and maximize outputs. Experience has shown that when surgeons lead in assessing new and emerging surgical techniques and technologies, the benefits of an evidence-based approach are realized, and the surgical community accepts the complementary role of evidence-based medicine in the provision of high-quality patient care.

The study of outcomes has become essential for guiding quality-of-care assessment and for clinical research. In this article, the properties and process of patient outcomes measurement are described. The limitations of traditional outcomes are discussed and contrasted with the emerging concept of "patient-centered" outcomes, measured by validated instruments to assess the effects of surgical interventions on health-related quality of life, functional status, pain, and patient satisfaction. The strengths and weaknesses of several measurement tools used in the surgical literature are evaluated. Finally, the authors introduce "composite outcomes" as a reflection of the multidimensional nature of modern patient care.

Evidence-based medicine, although ostensibly concerned with the research evidence underlying claims of efficacy for surgical procedures, has a direct connection with the ethics of surgical decision-making. Questions of whether new procedures should ever be performed on patients outside of a formal research protocol, what the patient should be told about the uncertainties inherent in the use of nonvalidated innovative procedures, when formal evaluation is necessary, what form that evaluation should take, and how the burdens and results of such research can be distributed fairly all involve balancing competing ethical principles. Good ethics requires good facts, and evidence from well-controlled experiments provides best information upon which to base decisions in these areas and to build ethical surgical practice.

> Evidence-based medicine provides a well-developed framework for evaluation of clinical research. Well-designed and adequately-powered randomized controlled trials provide the best information on therapeutic efficacy; however, extrapolation of the trials' conclusions to individual patients may be difficult, and for many important surgical problems, trial data are unavailable. A complementary approach of inferential decision-making helps address these limitations, and increases the clinician's confidence in the safety of an approach of unknown efficacy. Experience establishes norms and expectations, and emphasizes events that are uncommon but clinically important. Although it cannot eliminate uncertainty or controversy, the integration of analytic techniques of evidence, inference, and experience provides the surgeon with the best means of adapting treatment to the unique circumstances of the individual patient.

FORTHCOMING ISSUES

RECENT ISSUES

The Clinics are now available online!

www.theclinics.com

SURGICAL
CLINICS OF
NORTH AMERICA

ELSEVIER
SAUNDERS

Surg Clin N Am 86 (2006) xv–xviii

Foreword

Evidence-Based Surgery

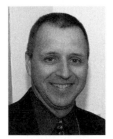

Ronald F. Martin, MD
Consulting Editor

Study your Physics well, and you'll be shown
In not too many pages that your art's good
Is to follow Nature insofar as it can.

—Dante, *The Inferno*

What do we know and how do we know it? This issue of the *Surgical Clinics of North America* by Dr. Jonathan Meakins and his colleagues may address the most important issue that we consider—how is it that we ascertain the truth? The truth, or at least our perception of it, is an elusive concept at best. It becomes even more elusive if one turns to the literature to ascertain it. One merely needs to pick up a journal from 20 or 30 years ago to realize that the amount of material contained within its pages has a wide variability in its persistence of representing the truth.

The evidence-based movement has suggested to us that if we apply rigorously scrutinized data collected in a randomized prospective fashion that we will be able to answer most, if not all, important clinical questions. Furthermore, if we follow the logical conclusion of converting this data into "best practices," we will eliminate bad outcomes. Although this notion has a sort of visceral appeal, it is probably far from the complete truth. One can certainly make the argument that under like circumstances, highly controlled algorithms and procedures should lend like outcomes. Unfortunately, we as surgeons face some unique challenges in this regard. Frequently, the nature of our profession causes us to deal with some issues that are not highly controllable, including time constraints, varying local referral patterns, diagnostic equipment, patient expectation, and, most notably, ourselves. Try

doi:10.1016/j.suc.2005.12.002   *surgical.theclinics.com*

though we may to deny it, the fact remains that we surgeons are in a competitive business—literally. Money, power, and prestige are at stake.

To borrow a phrase from our mathematical brethren, some problems have an "extreme sensitive dependence on initial conditions." This, in theory, explains why some problems, such as weather, are notoriously difficult to model accurately. Algorithms are very useful when you already know with a high degree of confidence what is wrong—frequently less so when you do not. This notion may introduce another potential problem with our emphasis on outcomes as a measure of success when we may have an inability to really measure appropriateness of indication. Most Morbidity & Mortality conferences I have had the privilege to attend have yielded more cases for discussion from failure to understand indication than from failure to execute an established "best practice" for the erroneously presumed problem. It would seem that we as surgeons, in particular general surgeons, will be faced with problems that lend themselves well to clinical pathways (eg, screening for colon cancer) and those that do not (eg, acute abdominal pain). The line between the two may shift and blur, but it is unlikely to disappear.

The concept itself of "best practice" has some Orwellian overtones that should give cause for concern under the best of circumstances. Who decides what is best and for whom? The reader of this issue will be privy to a very thoughtful analysis of this particular question. We have to consider that in this query, like so many others in life, where one stands depends upon where one sits. The public thinks (and expects) that we in the health care industry are all working together in pursuit of the greater good. And perhaps we are. Professional societies and organizations may feel that they know what is best as may government organizations, third party payers or advocacy groups. The greater good, though, may be a more nebulous target than we would care to admit. Another problem with labeling something a "best practice" is that it implies that to deviate from this is to offer something less than best, nearly by definition, rather than different from best. I prefer the term "best current practice," because at least it leaves room for the notion that continued improvement is expected.

Other issues that confound us are the proprietary issues regarding evidence; who owns it, who controls it, how do we disseminate it, how do we correct it? If we view our literature and process of investigation as the "research and development" of our industry, then we have some fundamental questions to address. In any business, research and development is part of a functioning business plan. There are economic laws that govern how it is funded, reimbursed, what percentage of profits can be returned to finance it, and what profit needs to be derived from it to sustain it. Our current system has no such truly cohesive strategy. Nor do we have clear guidance from society as to how much economic and regulatory burden they are willing to assume to achieve such goals. What is clear at present is that the economic position of our health care system in the context of a larger societal picture is in need of revision. This has been highlighted by the recent decision of

General Motors Corporation to downsize its production capacity and employee workforce, largely because of the company's reported inability to continue to support its employee and retiree health care cost. It has been said that "as goes General Motors so goes America." If there is even some truth to that statement, we will need to drastically reconstruct our health care financing structure as part of a national economic plan. This would likely lead to conditions where changes in the cooperation and real-time sharing of financial and information resources between and among "competitors" will take on new meaning.

The current dissemination of information is largely conducted through professional societies, their meetings and publications, and review publications such as this series. Historically, this has been a fairly effective and efficient process, although anyone who has been involved with these entities realizes that certain biases are inherent within the system that are barriers to incorporating and disseminating some evidence. The widely available access of electronic digital communications coupled with the advantage of worldwide instant communication may change this model. With this change we can expect the same occurrences as the print and television media industries have seen with internet-based information services and bloggers. These sites will have varying degrees of adherence to "rules of evidence" and the same (if not better) soapbox as the traditional journals have stood upon. A grass roots movement taking control of providing the framework for investigation and dissemination of information may seem unlikely—and perhaps it is, given some of the aspects of human investigation. But even IBM acknowledged the open-source APACHE project that provides the server software that our cultural infrastructure has come to largely depend upon was better developed by a collection of largely unrelated individuals than the mega-computing company could, or should, provide on its own. There is really no reason that I can see that we should consider ourselves substantially different in the broad strokes—and like IBM, other large professional organizations and societies will have to maintain a delicate balance between vigilant peer review and suppression of creative inquiry and development. First and foremost, we will all need to strive for what best serves the public. That debate, which will need to include the public in a meaningful way, has not yet occurred.

The evidence-based concept of surgery is a beginning and not an end to itself. Without some ability to organize our degree of confidence in the information that we have, we cannot reasonably expect to acquire, filter, absorb, or differentiate the torrent of data that presently flows toward us. The evidence-based rules cannot and will not supplant the need for inquiry, judgment, and personal caring that we as surgeons need to employ every day. We cannot eliminate all variability in surgical care and we cannot all be above average. The logical end point of all this effort is to allow us to bring to bear the full weight of what is available to help the individual patient with whom we are charged with being individually responsible for when he or she is ill. That has not changed—yet. The surgeon will remain the "transmission" or, if you prefer a more current metaphor, the "interface" between our collective professional wisdom and the patient. It is my hope that the reader of this issue will become better prepared to analyze our product and to critically assess our knowledge.

Ronald F. Martin, MD
Department of Surgery
Marshfield Clinic
1000 North Oak Avenue
Marshfield, WI 54449, USA

E-mail address: martin.ronald@marshfieldclinic.org

SURGICAL
CLINICS OF
NORTH AMERICA

ELSEVIER
SAUNDERS

Surg Clin N Am 86 (2006) xix–xxvi

Prologue

Evidence-Based Surgery—Inevitable?

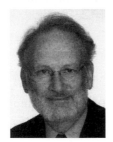 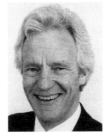

Jonathan L. Meakins, OC, MD, DSc,
FRCS(Hon), FRCS(C,Glas)

Sir Muir Gray, CBE, DSc, MD,
FRCP, FRCPS(Glas)

Guest Editors

Knowledge is the enemy of disease. This phrase appears on 30,000 pencils distributed by the National Electronic Library for Health, knowledge resource of the British National Health Service. This idea is at the very center of evidence-based surgery (EBS) and evidence-based surgical practice (EBSP). The knowledge to solve most clinical problems exists. The application of what we know already will have a bigger impact on health and disease than any drug or technology likely to be introduced in the next decade. Where we fail is often in not applying what is known. This may be as simple as a small clinical problem or as complex as the efficient and effective organization of a patient's journey through a surgical service. In most clinical situations, we know what should be done and also the best way in which to deliver the required clinical care. Yet we do not always succeed. Indeed, the Institute of Medicine has cataloged a large series of errors and failures in our health care systems and has suggested that between 44,000 and 98,000 deaths are the result of medical error. This indicates that knowledge was available but not applied.

Health care systems around the world are being heavily criticized for costing too much and not applying available resources effectively. A significant component of cost savings would be realized if best practices defined in medical, surgical, or hospital literature were universally adopted. Why is day case inguinal hernia repair or laparoscopic cholecystectomy not applied universally? The medical, surgical, anesthetic, nursing, and pain (symptom) control requirements are well known. The systems that permit delivery of these operations on a daily basis are well described. Every part of the patient journey is understood. Yet it has not happened as universally in the western world as one would expect. In the United States, insurance companies drive the agenda. In globally funded health care systems, failure to implement daily case work is not lack of knowledge but is a managerial, system, and professional failure. Knowledge management is integrating knowledge and its application.

The application of what we know can prevent or minimize ubiquitous systemic problems in health care:

- Medical error
- Uneven health care quality
- Inefficient use of resources
- Poor patient experience
- Overenthusiastic adoption of interventions of low or unproven value
- Failure to get new evidence into practice
- Variations in policy and practice

While each of the above requires a different bit of knowledge; each has a base of intellectual capital to enhance or resolve the difficulty. Knowing what we do know allows us to define what is really important: what we don't know. It is then possible to either find the information or perform the studies that will resolve the issues. The principles of patient safety and quality of patient-centered outcomes will be significantly enhanced by application of what we know to resolve the above list of health care deficiencies.

What is knowledge? There is no single universally accepted meaning, but a useful definition is that *data* are transformed into *information*, which is stored until someone wants to use it and *knowledge* is information in action.

In the context of EBS and EBSP, there are three types of knowledge:

- evidence (knowledge from research);
- statistics (knowledge from measurement of outcomes); and
- judgement (knowledge from experience).

This last is the sum of analysis of complications, morbidity, mortality, adverse events, and can be paraphrased as "good judgement comes from experience, and experience comes from bad judgement."

On August 22, 2005, a Google search using *evidence based surgery* provided 942,081 results, while a search using *evidence-based surgery* provided 343,950 results. Ask Jeeves provided 1,356,000 and 324,200 results, respectively, highlighting significantly the importance of defining our terms and our questions.

Further refinement to *evidence-based surgical practice* provided 183,534 (Google) and 105,500 (Ask Jeeves) results. On PubMed, *EBS* had 8666 articles, *E-BS* 2985, and *E-BSP* 950. The definition of terms is not only key to searching for information and evidence but also essential to its communication and implementation.

Objective

Our objective is to take the fishtail below and flesh out the skeleton highlighting where EBS and knowledge management can contribute to the delivery of high-value EBSP (Fig. 1).

Defining our terms

> A rose is a rose is a rose.
> —Gertrude Stein
> What's in a name? That which we call a rose
> By any other word would smell as sweet.
> —William Shakespeare, *Romeo and Juliet*
> "When I use a word", Humpty Dumpty said, in rather a scornful tone,
> "it means just what I choose it to mean—neither more nor less."
> —Lewis Caroll, *Through the Looking-Glass*

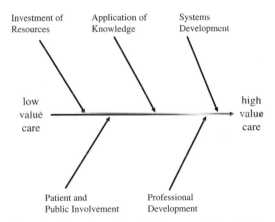

Fig. 1. Fishtail used to determine where EBS can contribute to high-value EBSP.

Visualize, if you will, Newcastle General Hospital, the hub of hospital care in the northeast for many years—solid, Victorian, dependable. The hospital's honest, uncompromising and practical atmosphere might strike you as an unlikely setting for the twentieth century's most influential philosopher, but Ludwig Wittgenstein was employed as a laboratory technician there during the Second World War. He showed such great promise as a laboratory investigator that attempts were made to persuade him to take up a scientific career. However, he chose to return to philosophy, linguistic philosophy in particular:

- proposing, in his tantalizing prose, that arguments and differences of opinion resulted from a failure to recognize that the two sides were using the same word with different meanings.

Defining words by words

The definition of a word is the summary of its meaning by a lexicographer such as Dr. Johnson, sometime Fellow of Pembroke College, Oxford, and compiler of the first great English dictionary. It was another Fellow of an Oxford College, Dr. James Murray, first Editor of the *Oxford English Dictionary*, who decided that a dictionary should contain not only definitions but also the meanings of the words by providing examples of the word in use, arranged chronologically to that the evolution of the meaning of the word could be understood. The meaning of a word is often different from its definition and can best be understood by observing its use. Murray's policy was at first fiercely resisted by some of the delegates of the Oxford University Press because of the effect this policy had on the magnitude, and therefore cost, of the exercise. Both were correct; the delegates because the task was immensely long (by the time of Murray's death 39 years after the commencement the dictionary had reached no further than the letter T), and Murray, because the enduring success of the *Oxford English Dictionary* has changed forever the way we think and find out about meanings.

Defining words by their usage

The principles of James Murray and the philosophy of Ludwig Wittgenstein are very similar. Wittgenstein's philosophy is difficult to read, and the two great works, the *Tractatus Logico Philosophicus* and *Philosophical Investigations*, consist of lean, numbered propositions, arranged hierarchically in the former and as a single sequence in the latter, but the absence of long paragraphs does not make them easy to understand. Easier access is provided by the numerous books about the twentieth century's most influential philosophers—for example, Antony Kenny's book *Wittgenstein*.

There is no meaning of a word that is always and indubitably the right meaning. There are only uses that are clear and uses that are not clear, uses that are new and uses that are not new. The need to observe how a word is used to understand its meaning is one of the principles of Wittgenstein's philosophy that underpins this book, and rather than expecting the reader to buy Last's *Dictionary of Epidemiology*, excellent though that is, we have endeavored to make it clear how we are using particular terms.

Two other of Wittgenstein's principles are also relevant to decision-makers:

- New words such as "Internet," or new uses of words such as "World Wide Web" can clarify, confuse and be useful, but as the term becomes more widely used by more people, its use becomes increasingly diverse, and there may come a point at which the term causes more confusion than clarity and should no longer be used. Consider, for example, how often you have heard the term "evidence" used when it was obvious that it was being used with a different meaning from the way in which you would use it.

- Many arguments—Wittgenstein believed all arguments—result from a failure to appreciate that the people involved have failed to agree on the meaning of the terms being used. Consider, for example, how often you have heard arguments about the proposition that "evidence-based medicine destroys clinical freedom" without time being taken to reach agreement on the terms "evidence-based medicine," "destroys," and "clinical freedom."

Decision-making can be improved and arguments prevented, therefore, by prefacing the debate with statements such as: "When we use the word "evidence," we mean "knowledge derived from research"; when we use knowledge derived from our own experience, we shall make that clear."

Word euthanasia

Sometimes it is necessary to take steps to discontinue the use of a term that is consistently and frequently the cause of confusion and as such prevents understanding and progress. This is less frequently necessary in management than in clinical practice because management decision-making involves many terms that are created and enter widespread use until they themselves become displaced by later fashions. *Benchmarking* and *modernizing* are examples of such terms, and the same fate may, heaven forfend, befall *evidence-based decision-making*, but if it does cause more confusion than clarity then it should be dropped from decision-making discourse. Even in clinical practice, however, terms can cause confusion and may need to be deleted from debate.

In his highly praised biography, Ray Monk describes how Wittgenstein, when a technician in a research laboratory in Guy's Hospital in 1941, formed a Medical Research Council team whose leader had observed that "there is in practice a wide variation in the application of the diagnosis of 'shock' without an agreed meaning of the term" that was harmful to patients and "renders it impossible to assess the efficacy of the various methods of treatment adopted." He argued that "there is good ground, therefore" for the view that it is better to avoid the diagnosis of "shock" and to replace it with an accurate and complete record of a patient's state and progress, together with the treatment given. We have been similarly unsuccessful with "sepsis." Only Humpty Dumpty really knows!

Wittgenstein was himself influenced by a physicist, Hertz, who proposed dropping the use of the term "force" from the vigorous debates of the time, accepting that if this were done "the questions as to the nature of force will not have been answered but our minds, no longer vexed, will cease to ask illegitimate questions." Wittgenstein, in paying homage to this approach, said that "in my way of doing philosophy, its whole aim is to give an expression such a form that certain disquietudes disappear." He also proposed that if Dr. Grant was required to include the word *shock* in his annual report, as some authorities wished, the word should be printed "upside down to emphasize its unsuitability."

There is no evidence that Wittgenstein studied the work of Murray, but he would surely have approved of his painstaking collection of examples of the word in use that are set out, clearly allowing Murray to take bundles of examples of the meanings in use, held together by a pin, so that he could "write and polish and fuss with and burnish, for each one of the words and senses and meanings, what he divined to be their definitions."

Defining words by numbers

Vienna at the end of the Hapsburg empire was in the final stages of its glory, already turning a little rotten on the bough. Although rottenness implies decay, decay is necessary for the creation of new life forms. Wittgenstein was a product of Vienna—or, to be more precise, of the intellectual and wealthy Jewish community living in Vienna; so, too, was Malinowski. Malinowski argued contrary to Wittgenstein that knowledge was created, not by the lonely intellectual sitting at his desk, as Wittgenstein did throughout the English winters, but by groups of people taking and using language to create new knowledge.

The Vienna School of Philosophy flourished as Wittgenstein left the city and became very influential, particularly in Britain, where it gave rise to what is known as *logical positivism*, the leading figure and most eloquent reporter of which was A.J. Ayer. In *Language, Truth and Logic,* Ayer took an approach to the definition of a term that did not rely on words at all. He proposed that instead of trying to understand the meaning of a proposition by analyzing the meaning of the individual terms that compose it, another approach should be taken.

"The criteria which we use to test the genuineness of apparent statements of fact is the criterion of verifiability. We say that a sentence is factually significant to any given person, if, and only if, he knows how to verify the propositions which it purports to express—that is, if he knows what observations would lead him, under certain conditions, to accept the proposition as being true, or reject it as being false. And with regard to questions the procedure is the same. We enquire in every case what observations would lead us to answer the question, one way or the other; and, if none can be discovered, we must conclude that the sentence under consideration does not, as far as we are concerned, express a genuine question, however strongly its grammatical appearance may suggest that it does."

The logical positivists believe that no term should be examined in isolation—a study of the term "efficiency" would be pointless—but investigated in the context of propositions, such as "this hospital is more efficient than that hospital." To define the meaning of this proposition, a logical positivist would not have recourse to a dictionary but instead seek to agree on the data that would need to be collected to confirm or refute it. Thus, for this particular proposition, the debate immediately becomes: "How would you measure efficiency?" Options include:

- cost per case;
- throughput per bed;
- percentage of costs spent on administration.

Meaning, reality, and language

The traditional view of language is that it describes reality. This is undoubtedly true for physical objects such as "a table" or "a chair," unless one belongs to the more skeptical school of philosophy, which holds that everything ceases to exist when one closes one's eyes. For social constructs, however, language does not simply describe reality; it creates it.

The clearest description of the relationship between language and reality comes from anthropologists, notably Benjamin Lee Whorf, who worked as a loss adjuster for The Hartford Fire Insurance Company and studied the language of the Hopi Indians. He created the theory of linguistic relativity, which proposes that language creates social realities such as "the future" or "the quality of evidence"—or, indeed, "evidence-based health care." Through the use and evolution of language comes social change and social reality. The work of the anthropologists such as Wharf and Edward Sapir, whose Wharf Sapir hypothesis of linguistic relativity is the best articulation of this concept, for example, in the statement that "the fact of the matter is that the 'real world' is to a large extent unconsciously built up on the language habits of the group" has been developed by sociologists. The most accessible sociologic text is *The Social Construction of Reality* by Berger and Luckman.

Words have meanings, but the meanings create and change reality as well as express it.

Indefinite definitions

Throughout this issue of the *Surgical Clinics of North America*, we have tried to give a clear definition of a term without implying that our definition is *the* definition; *caveat lector*, let the reader beware.

Jonathan L. Meakins, OC, MD, DSc, FRCS(Hon), FRCS(C,Glas)*
Sir Muir Gray, CBE, DSc, MD, FRCP, FRCPS(Glas)
Nuffield Department of Surgery, University of Oxford
John Radcliffe Hospital, Headington, Oxford OX3 9DU, UK
*Corresponding author

E-mail addresses: jonathan.meakins@nds.ox.ac.uk (J.L. Meakins);
muir.gray@dphpc.ox.ac.uk (M. Gray)

Further readings

Ayer AJ. Language, truth and logic. London: Penguin; 1936.

Berger PL, Luckman T. The social construction of reality. London: Routledge and Keegan; 1967.

Institute of Medicine. To err is human: building a safer health system. Washington, DC: Institute of Medicine; 1999.

Monk R. Wittgenstein. London: Vintage Press; 1991. p. 445–7.

Winchester S. The meaning of everything: the story of the Oxford English Dictionary. Oxford (UK): Oxford University Press; 2003.

ELSEVIER
SAUNDERS

Surg Clin N Am 86 (2006) 1–16

SURGICAL
CLINICS OF
NORTH AMERICA

Evidence-Based Surgery

Jonathan L. Meakins, OC, MD, DSc, FRCS(Hon), FRCS(C,Glas)

Nuffield Department of Surgery, John Radcliffe Hospital, University of Oxford, Headington, Oxford OX3 9DU, England, UK

Evidence-based medicine (EBM) has entered into the lexicography of clinical practice. We are here involved with that set of knowledge that relates to surgery, clearly a subset of medicine overall, and to surgical practice. The author will therefore substitute evidence-based surgery (EBS) for EBM and refer to its application clinically as evidence-based surgical practice (EBSP). EBSP should incorporate the entire patient journey from first contact to completion of the care episode whether short or long term.

The EBM proponents and gurus have had much scorn showered on them since the introduction of the term and the development of coherent processes for clinical application and a structure into which to place the approach. Established clinicians were ruffled at the very idea that their clinical practices were not evidence-based. Most considered themselves to be up-to-date, and some were opinion leaders in their field. The operative word is, of course, opinion. Our approach to any clinical problem is a reflection of our training, and our trainers, and often what we last read or listened to or even ignored.

What is evidence-based surgery?

Evidence-based surgery could be defined as the integration of: best research evidence (clinically relevant research, basic science, relating to diagnosis, treatment, prognosis) with clinical expertise (skills and experience adapted to a particular patient) and patient values (patient preference and attitudes to clinical entity and its overall management) [1].

The definition and the values it expresses are hard to dispute. The devil is in the details, however, and the most contentious and difficult of these are in clarifying, defining, or establishing "best research evidence." Typically, a single key paper in a recently published journal of high repute may carry the

E-mail address: jonathan.meakins@nds.ox.ac.uk

doi:10.1016/j.suc.2005.10.004
surgical.theclinics.com

day. The classic debating trick on rounds: "In this week's journal, X, not Y, is the way to manage this clinical scenario." Yet in reality, the best evidence is usually a summary of all the evidence that will assist solving the clinical problem with the elimination of bias. The detailed process for a simple question in a particular patient might be different from the same clinical problem in a population. The steps, however, are essentially the same:

1. Define the question.
2. Search for the evidence.
3. Critically appraise the literature.
4. Apply the results: on a patient or a population.
5. Evaluate the outcome.

Closing the circle—evaluation of outcome—is as important as any of the other steps.

There are specific tools that must be mastered to implement this approach to any clinical issue. Just as dissecting with a scalpel is a learned skill and somewhat different from using Metzenbaum scissors, search methodology has multiple techniques that one can use to identify the same collection of articles. Multiple techniques can be learned, but as with most tools, a favorite approach or technique will emerge. Searching is an important tool to recognize and use well.

The next key tool is critical appraisal. This does not mean evaluation of the center (reputable), the authors (well-known to me or by reputation) or the level of agreement of the conclusions with our preformed and often well-established thoughts. It means using a structured framework to evaluate the literature (evidence). When asking a question relating to a specific patient and clinical problem [2], the article must address three questions:

1. Is the evidence from this randomized, controlled trial (RCT) valid?
2. If valid, is it important?
3. When valid and important, can it be applied to the patient or problem at hand?

We must always separate the statistically significant from the clinically important. Box 1 provides the template for evaluating an article and facilitates its use in answering the above three questions:

A useful concept to calculate from the critical appraisal is the number needed to treat (NNT). The NNT is the number of patients treated to achieve the primary goal in a patient. For surgeons deciding upon an operation; the number needed to harm (NNH) is as important, and ought to be integrated into any clinical or operative decision [1].

In their article on finding and appraising evidence elsewhere in this issue, McCulloch and Badenoch outline the creation of a critically appraised topic or CAT. This is another tool of great use, because once done it can be updated as new evidence surfaces. Most approaches to CAT making and application of results do depend on a number of statistical calculations.

Box 1. Guidelines for appraising a therapeutic article

1. Did the authors answer the question?
2. Were groups of patients randomized?
3. Are the comparison groups similar?
4. Were patients blinded?
5. Was it placebo-controlled?
6. Was evaluation of effect blinded?
7. Was the length of study appropriate?
8. What was the follow-up rate?
9. Are there clear measures of outcome?
10. Was it an "intention-to-treat" trial?
11. Is the context of the study similar to your own?
12. Did the treatment work?

Adapted from Dawes M. Randomized controlled trials. In: Evidence-Based Practice: A primer for Health Care Professionals. (eds. Dawes M. et al. Churchill Livingstone, London) 1999; p. 52.

Table 1 lists some of the terms to define outcomes and used to calculate measures of the importance of findings. To be clear, if the NNT to benefit from an operation were 30 and NNH were also 30, serious consideration to nonoperative therapy would be appropriate. The chance of benefit is low and equal to that of harm. If the NNT were 5, thinking might be very different.

The terms listed in Table 1 seem daunting and a trifle irritating, but they do assist in understanding the final assessment of the value of an intervention [3]. Systematic reviews and meta-analyses as well as results of clinical trials will use these terms to clarify the magnitude of a treatment effect or its absence.

Table 1
Measures of outcome and useful terms

ARR	Absolute risk reduction
CER	Control event rate
CI	Confidence interval
EER	Experimental event rate
OR	Odds ratio
QALY	Quality-adjusted life-year
ROC	Receiver-operating characteristic
RR	Relative risk
RRR	Relative reduction in risk

Adapted from Dawes M. Randomised controlled trials. In: Dawes M, Davies P, Gray A, et al. Evidence-based practice: a primer for health care professionals. London: Churchill Livingstone; 1999. p. XI.

An integral component of EBM/EBS is the hierarchy of evidence. The table in the article by Burger, Sugarmen, and Goodman on ethical issues elsewhere in this issue outlining the levels of evidence and grades of recommendation is from the Centre for Evidence-Based Medicine at the University of Oxford [1,4]. Although in general surgeons are concerned with therapy and its effects, the table also outlines the various types of evidence associated with prognosis, diagnosis, and economic analysis. The studies are stratified into levels of evidence by their quality, lack of bias, homogeneity, and so forth. There are five levels. The strongest evidence, 1a, is a systematic review of RCTs with homogeneity. The weakest is expert opinion, however qualified. The level identifies the quality of the evidence and leads to a grade of recommendation A through D. The development of the levels of evidence and grades of recommendation has been iterative [4–7].

The levels of evidence most available to surgeons and operative therapy are listed in Table 2.

Most of the surgical literature consists of case series and has been heavily criticized for the absence of RCTs and well-structured prospective studies [8,9]. There is nonetheless a significant body of information in the literature that has directed therapy of common and uncommon clinical problems. Management of that knowledge and identification of significant lacuna via critical appraisal is a way forward.

Is surgical practice evidence-based?

The surgical community's answer will inevitably be "of course." Two studies have specifically addressed the question.. Howes and colleagues [10] evaluated surgical treatment to sequential emergency admissions and found that their practice was supported by Level I evidence in 24% and Level II in 71%. These were common problems and evaluation was of overall treatment plans. The second study [11] retrospectively assessed all admissions to a general surgical service, identified diagnosis and treatment, and then found supporting evidence in the literature for management. The studies were not classified by level and quality of RCTs was not defined. The distribution of study quality is similar to that of the above study, but at least 30% are Level III, grade C or lower quality studies. Although it is possible to find some support for most therapies, disciplined critical appraisal of the

Table 2
Levels of evidence

Grade	Level	
A	1c	All or none
B	2a	Systematic review of cohort studies
B	2b	A cohort study
B	2c	"Outcomes" research
C	4	Case series
D	5	Expert opinion

studies may demonstrate significant flaws, structural biases, or failure of adequate follow-up. The surgical literature has been criticized [8,9,12]; the medical literature in general is often seen to be flawed through poor studies, editorial bias, poor peer review, the power of industry, lack of generalizability, and many more weaknesses. Indeed, it seems hard to believe that we depend so much on a body of knowledge that is so heavily criticized. Critical appraisal, systematic reviews, and meta-analysis will help to identify the value of knowledge that we have and that which we require.

Despite some support of the notion that surgical practice is evidence-based, there are significant data that suggest it is not. Examples follow of demonstrated failure to apply grade A recommendations. The use and timing of prophylactic antibiotics for prevention of wound infection (surgical site infection [SSI]) following an operation has been clearly defined for decades. Yet an important factor in SSIs is the failure to use perioperative antibiotics correctly. Classen and colleagues [13] identified inappropriate antibiotic prophylactic in the mid 1980s.

The Latter Day Saints (LDS) Hospital in Salt Lake City, Utah has tracked appropriate use of prophylactic antibiotics from 1985 through 1998. The use of education, and specifically a computer reminder system, improved the appropriate administration of antibiotics from 40% to 96% over a period of 6 years. When the reminders were discontinued, compliance dropped to 80%. Appropriate use was 97% to 99% upon reintroduction of the system [14].

In what must have been part of the same system, a computer-assisted management program for antibiotic use improved quality of patient care and reduced costs [14].

There are areas of surgical practice in colorectal surgery in which the data are solid regarding use of drains, antibiotic prophylaxis, and use of subcutaneous heparin to prevent thromboembolic complications of an operation. Indeed, no one could pass the "Principles of Surgery" examination before board certification without knowledge of these three data sets. Despite everyone knowing how best to use the evidence on these three issues, Wasey and coworkers [15] have demonstrated clearly on a colorectal service.

Overuse of drains
Underuse of heparin
Misuse of antibiotics (timing, duration)

We know what to do, yet somehow fail to manage and implement the knowledge we have [16].

Recent systemic reviews and meta-analysis of the use of drains [17] in abdominal surgery and of nasogastric tubes [18] in general surgery have confirmed individual studies showing absence of patient benefit and the possibility of harm. Yet a tour on any general surgical floor and some others will confirm that both abdominal drains and nasogastric tubes are in common use. Why?

Further evidence that we know what to do but often fail to implement that knowledge is presented by Dexter and colleagues [19]. They evaluated the use of computer reminders for the use of aspirin following a myocardial infarction, prophylactic heparin, and vaccination, influenza or pneumococcal, in defined clinical settings. The indications for these interventions are well-known. Yet for the vaccines, use was about 1% without reminders and only 36% or 51% with them. For heparin and aspirin post-discharge, use was increased to one third from 19% and 28% respectively. Some physicians routinely ignored the reminders, others were responsive. Yet if asked, most would acknowledge that there was a valid evidence base for these simple interventions.

Evidence-based surgical practice: why is it so difficult?

There are a number of more or less defensible reasons, associated both with surgical practice and the nature of surgeons, that explain the difficulties, and a number of less defensible reasons for why there is so much variation in the management of specific clinical problems. More difficult is understanding geographical variations in the performance of specific procedures. In this instance, the author will not approach the regional variations, but the concepts are likely to be much the same as they are when details of operative and postoperative management are examined and found to vary significantly within an institution as well as across institutions. A major driver for variations in clinical practice relates to the surgical training structure, which is essentially an apprentice-based approach through which surgical trainees are expected to practice in the model of their teachers. If therefore there are four colorectal surgeons on a service and all do a particular component of patient preparation, operative practice, or postoperative management differently, trainees will do what each surgeon instructs and eventually develop some synthesis to manage their own patients. Thus the surgical training structure dictates a major variation in clinical practice.

There is also a question of what is acceptable evidence. The process in Australia for the evaluation of new techniques or new technology is outlined in the article by Maddern elsewhere in this issue. Many of the Australian evaluative processes end up indicating that more research is required. In many instance, this remains the case in sorting aspects of surgical evidence, and can be seen not only in the Australian Safety and Efficacy Register of New Internventional Procedures-Surgical (ASERNIP–S) process but also that of the Cochrane collaboration. In many instances in which we take very dogmatic approaches, a systematic review will indicate that the data are not available to support any of them. This may mean that it does not matter how a particular problem is approached, or that there is a best method but we may not like it.

Frequently, there are areas in which best practice has been identified—for example the use of drains, postoperative pain management, or nasogastric tubes—yet variation is common. A major problem is that implementation of a single approach supported by the evidence will require significant change in professional behavior, which is a particularly irksome administrative task for leader and follower. It tends to impact on professionals' belief in the autonomy of their clinical decisions and their right to make specific defined approaches to the management of their own patients. Change is hard; changing a professional's practice is really hard. The translation of knowledge to practice has foundered on a profession's culture [20,21].

A final consideration regarding defensibility is that rules of evidence are sometimes not useful for procedural-based problems. There are many aspects in surgery that are quite suitable to an RCT; there are others much less so, and this subject is addressed subsequently.

Much less defensible are the attitudes that it is "my way or the highway," and that personal experience indicates best practice. One hears remarks that the author or the journal is not credible. The reluctance to change is enormous, and the resistance such that a negotiation over relatively simple clinical protocols becomes lost in dogma and is often compounded by the absence of critical evidence. The worst arguments are those where the evidence is sparse. The dogmatism has a religious fervor. One must, however, ask the question: If it doesn't matter, why can the same problem not be managed by everyone in the same manner? The benefits to nursing, house staff, costs, patient safety, and so on would be great. The most obvious example around which there are considerable differences of opinion, despite the presence of good evidence, is the use of drains or nasogastric tubes in association with gastrointestinal surgery. If drains are associated with increased complications without particular benefit to the patient, it would seem a simple matter of eliminate their use [17], yet this has proved to be an irksome problem, a good example of which is the use of abdominal drains in open cholecystectomy. Studies were done as to whether the drain should be through a separate stab wound or come out the wound, but in reality, every study looking at the value of those drains in cholecystectomy indicated that they were of no benefit to the patient and actually had a clinically significant complication rate as well as occupying nursing time and occupying doctor time. On ward rounds, the question is posed: Should the drain come out? "Well, it is draining a little bit, perhaps we will leave it for another day," and so on. The story with nasogastric tubes is the same [19]. It seems obvious that a group should arrive at a standard policy where neither of these instruments was used except in defined circumstances, yet this has proven to be exceptionally difficult to achieve. The reasons have to do with tradition (it is traditional to do this or, in my training program, that is how we did it), and a conflict in belief (we don't believe the study because we can remember a situation in which X or Y was useful). To submit all patients to something that has a small benefit in a small group of patients and yet has complications that are measurable in the larger group, seems madness. It is here that use of the NNT and NNH can be very useful.

Finally, the concept of understanding who is the patient is important. Frequently interventions are used because the surgeon is worried. Putting a drain in the patient to relieve surgeon anxiety does not seem to be an appropriate therapy for either the surgeon's anxiety or the patient's operation. It is important to recognize that in every doctor–patient relationship there are indeed two parties or patients:

(1) the patient who is receiving medical advice or therapy
(2) the physician who is concerned that what he does for the patient is in the patient's best interest, and who makes sometimes decisions on the basis of personal angst.

It is important to suppress the need of physicians to look after their concerns and apply best evidence to patient care. A common example of surgeon worry dictating a decision is prolonging the use of prophylactic antibiotics. The reasoning being: "That was a difficult operation, we better give three days of antibiotics," despite the dangers of resistance and *Clostridium difficile*, and the large body of evidence that there is no patient benefit.

In the long run, a major concern must be that if the profession does not use best evidence, external pressures will force the issue [16,20,21].

What would be the face of evidence-based surgical practice?

The most obvious change, perhaps the unacceptable one, would be standardization of pre- and postoperative care. Evidence-based protocols and care maps would be standard operating practice.

In some instances, it would be the recognition that many details of care do not really matter that much, and when evidence is not available it should be possible to arrive at some reasonable compromise that is suitable for simplifying modern surgical practice, the patient's journey, and outcomes. Very good examples would be "When do you remove clips following an open operation?" and "Should that be done in hospital or at home?" With the shortening of patient stay in hospital, sutures or clips are frequently left in place to be removed subsequently. Perhaps it would be more suitable to remove them in hospital and apply adhesive strips, or to close the wound in another manner, such as a subcuticular stitch with absorbable sutures, steristrips in the operating room, or tissue glues that are recently being promoted by industry. It should surely be possible to arrive at an agreement in a service as to how to manage such a simple issue, yet it seems to be very difficult.

There are nonetheless many processes of care that can be protocolized on the basis of very good evidence. Henrik Kehlet has developed such a program in Copenhagen relating to what is termed "fast-track surgery" [22,23]. This is in essence a variation of a care map or protocolized surgery. At the heart of this approach is a common pathway for therapy that is developed by all relevant health care professionals and is composed of evidence-based elements. Where data are not available, team agreements are established. Checklists and care maps are integral to these patient management approaches. Monitoring of outcomes is important. Indeed, the process is identical to the five steps of EBS identified at the beginning of this article. The evaluation step allows, perhaps guarantees, continuous quality improvement. Patient education is a key component and makes the patient an integrated participant. The system can plan patient discharge following a colon resection on the third postoperative day [23].

The fast-track approach has been applied to a number of procedures, including aortocoronary bypass and joint replacements of the hip and knee. Although the development of these programs requires considerable energy and flattening of the clinical hierarchy, they can be achieved. The evidence suggests that the clinical outcomes are more than satisfactory [23]. Failure of wide adoption of these approaches speaks in part to the fact that it is difficult, and that a traditional clinical approach that appears to work is very difficult to modify.

Cardiac surgeons have been exposed to publication of their results in the popular press. It is uncertain if this has led to significant improvement in regional results or transfer of high-risk patients elsewhere. An approach to registry data, evidence, and continuous quality improvement has been demonstrated by the Northern New England Cardiovascular Disease Study Group (NNECVDSG). They have demonstrated shortened length of stay, reduced costs, and improved outcome with a judicious mix of their own risk-adjusted data and application of best evidence. All six units in the NNECVDSG have demonstrated benefits, and all have contributed to improved outcomes [24–26].

Are there external drivers?

External drivers to push clinical practice toward a more standardized EBSP (perhaps the term "best practice" ought to be used) are principally three. First, the cost of health care throughout the Western world is increasing almost exponentially and needs to be managed. Second, issues surrounding patient safety have highlighted the reality that there are vast differences in the way in which similar problems are handled, and that undoubtedly some will not matter; however, in many areas it is likely that there will be a best practice approach, and it is up to the medical profession to sort these out. Third, a threatening medico-legal environment, increasing in all Organization for Economic Cooperation and Development (OECD) countries, is using concepts of evidence-based practice and standardized approaches to the management of common problems to support claims. In circumstances in which there is an untoward event, failure to have used best evidence leaves the clinician open to legal liability.

Patient safety has been highlighted in recent years following the publication of the Institute of Medicine's report *To Err is Human* [27]. This was followed by a second report entitled *Crossing the Quality Chasm* [28]. Following publication of the first, newspaper headlines across North America reported that 44,000 to 98,000 deaths a year were the result of medical error. Although these are estimates, they nonetheless caught the attention of policy makers, government, and patient advocacy groups, as well as the medico-legal fraternity. Patient safety issues are therefore very high on the agenda of a knowledge-management conscious profession. In the United Kingdom, the *Times of London* recently headlined "Blundering hospitals kill 40,000 every year" [29]. That over 50% of medical errors are pharmacological does not leave procedure-based medicine in the clear. Errors in hospital are either those of omission or commission if one excludes technical complications or complications associated with patient disease or comorbidity. If there is an error of omission or commission, there is a knowledge base against which decisions can be tested either preoperatively, operatively, or postoperatively. It is coordination of those evidence bases that are required, and their application rather more routinely to common problems. Recognizing that this interferes with physician autonomy, the issues of patient safety will not long tolerate the desire for professional independence versus continuous quality improvement evidence-based surgical care.

It is likely that some of the solutions will be modeled after the airline industry, which has defined the importance of checklists as well as persistent and ongoing cross-checking. This demands a flattening of the traditional hierarchy present in surgical practice, in which junior members of the teams or nonphysicians are unwelcome in the identification of problems. There is indeed evidence that the flattening of the hierarchy is beneficial, as demonstrated in pediatric cardiac surgery through the work of Professor de Leval and colleagues [30]. Some of the solutions will incorporate the use of checklists in the operating room, where the surgical team, the anesthetist, and the nursing team all agree on the name of the patient, the operation to be done, the site and side of the operation, whether or not antibiotics have been given or are to be given, the use of heparin for thromboembolic prophylaxis, the presence of a catheter, and the presence or absence of drains, tubes, and techniques of pain control in the postoperative period. The checklist would be adapted to procedure and discipline, incorporating other relevant details.

The medical profession in all developed countries is feeling increasingly threatened by malpractice suits. The EBM movement has touched the legal profession as it uses the evidence to question medical practice when there has been an adverse event. The two Institute of Medicine (IOM) reports further identifying medical errors and issues of patient safety have used data to support their contentions [27,28]. If evidence-based practice is to become the standard of care rather than local practice, not an unreasonable scenario, the surgical profession must learn EBS and EBSP [29].

How should surgical innovation be assessed?

Surgical innovation falls roughly into two categories. The first relates to techniques and technology, all of which are tied into the development of new procedures or modification of old procedures. One must always ask the question "How should a new operation or a new technique, or the use of a new technology, be introduced into clinical practice?" The other major area of surgical innovation relates to processes of care, including the previously mentioned fast-track approaches, care maps, and the development and use of clinical guidelines. All of these require assessment and evaluation and, in many instances, the question needs to be posed "Are the rules of evidence different for surgical procedures or aspects of surgical innovation that involve clinical care?" The standard approach for assessment of any clinical entity has been the RCT, preferably double-blind. One needs to pose the question of what is the role of the RCT in evaluation and new procedures and new technology, as well as innovative approaches to processes of care [32].

If we look at the clinical advances in techniques and systems of care associated with aortocoronary bypass, hepatic resection, pancreatic resection, or aortic surgery for aneurysm disease, incremental changes in clinical care have been too small to measure, yet despite operating in increasingly complex clinical circumstances, morbidity and mortality in association with all of these procedures has declined over time. This is undoubtedly associated in some part with improved surgical technique; however, the sum of tiny improvements in staging, surgical approaches, aspects of operating room technology, and advances in anesthetic care, pain management, and all aspects of postoperative management are responsible. There is indeed some evidence that results improve over time as an individual surgeon develops an operative team and the team approach to management of a specific operation. This is often ascribed to the surgeon and the surgeon's technique, but is almost certainly related to a comprehensive and coordinated approach understood by the team [30,33]. We see knowledge management, EBSP, in action.

One of the critical issues in evaluating surgical innovation, either of systems or related to procedures, has been the nature of the study required to demonstrate progress. The majority of surgical studies are observational in one manner or another and the number of RCTs is seen to be too low [8]. Box 2 outlines some of the progress areas in surgery where RCTs have either been not required, not helpful or, indeed, have been the keys to understanding progress. There is no question that observational studies can provide very important information in the evaluation of new techniques, and in some instances, will not allow for the performance of an RCT, for a variety of reasons frequently outlined [32,34]. Arguments have recently been made to indicate that the circumstances in which RCTs are not suitable in surgical situations are plentiful, and pleas have been made for other forms of evaluative techniques to be applied to develop the evidence base defining technical approaches to a variety of issue [32,34,35]. Box 3 outlines some of the difficulties in surgical RCTs, but also highlights that there are educational problems that surgeons can easily address to rectify some of these issues. The establishment of an educational approach to clinical epidemiology with

---

Box 2. Progress areas in surgery

Procedures in which RCTs are helpful
- Extracranial-intracranial (EC-IC) bypass
- Carotid endarterectomy
- Lung reduction surgery
- Stenting of vessels
- Breast cancer surgical trials
- Colon cancer adjuvant therapy

Procedures in which RCTs are not helpful
- Percutaneous drainage
- Liver transplantation
- Laparoscopic adrenalectomy or splenectomy
- Inflammatory bowel disease

RCTs not required
- "The penicillin effect"
- Hip replacement
- Liver resection for colorectal metastases
- Nonoperative management of splenic injury
- Drainage of subphrenic abscess

---

the acquisition of the discipline's tools, many of which are incorporated in the principles of EBS, should allow a satisfactory evidence-based approach to be developed.

The evolution of interventional radiology and the inevitable competition that is surfacing between surgical practice and the ability of radiologists to perform similar procedures in a minimally invasive manner will drive comparative studies to be established. An example recently published is that of the International Subarachnoid Aneurysm trial, in which it was demonstrated that the use of coils via interventional neuroradiologists provided a better outcome to patients who had cerebral vascular aneurysms than did an

---

Box 3. Difficulties in surgical RCTs

- Equipoise: patients/surgeons
- Bias: selection and observer
- Blinding
- Learning curve—when
- Effectiveness versus efficacy
- Standardization of technique
- Lack of education in clinical epidemiology

---

open surgical approach [36]. There will be increasing studies of this sort, and these are of course suitable for RCTs to define which is the best approach. The standards required to ensure that comparable groups and techniques are being compared will continue to be difficult. Nevertheless it is obvious that procedures can be compared. The majority of studies evaluating surgery have been comparisons to best medical management, the surgical procedure having been established as safe and effective via observational studies or cohort studies.

Although the difficulties in RCTs have been identified in the past [32,34,35], it is useful to point out that some of these are quite significant (see Box 3). The equipoise required to do a procedure-based RCT is significant. It is required on the part of both the patient and the surgeon. When conducting an RCT of laparoscopic cholecystectomy, it became quickly apparent that the patients did not have equipoise with respect to the procedure. Patients had been sufficiently biased that their wish was to have the "minimally invasive approach." Not long after patients lost their equipoise, surgeons did as well. The study had to be terminated [37]. In addition, bias with respect to patient selection and observer evaluation is a significant variable in this setting, and blinding both patient and evaluator to procedure done can be quite difficult. When during the learning curve should the RCT be done? The learning curve can be quite protracted in some procedures, those of a complex technical or skill level, whereas others are complex as a result of the entire team requiring training in the production of standardized results [30,33]. There is the question of effectiveness versus efficacy. That is, in the hands of a master surgeon, what would the results be compared with those of surgeons representing average ability in the community. Standardization of technique is enormously difficult, as is seen in the recent Veteran's Administration study of laparoscopic versus open hernia repair [38]. Continuous monitoring was required to ensure that both operations were done in a completely standardized manner. It is almost inevitable that surgeons will constantly modify their techniques and thereby create difficulties with the result to the end point. Finally, a part of the problem within surgery relates to a lack of education in the clinical tools of clinical epidemiology.

All of this having been said, it is the surgeon's responsibility to define the evidence base upon which our clinical practice is founded, and some of these issues will need to be faced up to squarely.

What are some of the solutions?

Driving forces have already been mentioned with respect to the need for EBSP. These drivers will demand for all surgeons an understanding of the principles of EBS and how to implement them in practice. The objective is not standardization of all aspects of surgical clinical activity, but to ensure that patients at all times receive optimal surgical care. Therefore, from a surgical career point of view, understanding the issues associated with surgical epidemiology, knowledge management, and EBSP has implications for clinicians in the community, surgeons in large metropolitan hospitals, surgeon scholars, and the academic surgeon. All need to have some understanding of not only the evaluation of the evidence and how to find it but, in addition, application of those concepts to continuous quality improvement and closing a circle of surgical audit. These issues are well outlined by Jones [31] and in his American Surgical Association Presidential Address. If the surgical profession has an obligation to redefine clinical modus operandi and educational processes, the arguments for formal training in aspects of clinical epidemiology during the surgical residency program are obvious, because all surgeons will benefit from those educational exercises.

What would be required from the surgical community to implement EBSP and the concepts of continuous quality improvement, which are innately linked with the knowledge management required, is leadership within the discipline for the cultural changes required. In addition, surgical training needs to be modified to be less apprentice-associated and less individualistic in the solution of problems, and leadership is required to identify what matters and what doesn't matter.

Surgical societies can contribute effectively in the way in which their annual programs and continuing professional development aspects are developed by insisting on specific standards with respect to the studies presented. Journals, in addition, have a specific responsibility to ensure through peer review and editorial assessment that published articles meet certain standards. In addition, a number of journals, including the *Canadian Journal of Surgery*, the *Journal of the American College of Surgeons*, and the *British Journal of Surgery* have either classified their articles or have specific segments of the journal that address evidence-based principles.

Further work can be done through large surgical organizations such as the American College of Surgeons, which has developed a clinical trials operation most obviously seen through the American College of Surgeons Oncology Group, but is also seen in the recent studies in hernia repair—comparison of techniques, as well as evaluation of watchful waiting [36]. The College, in addition, has a research and optimal patient care division as one of its principle enterprises and this is outlined in the article by Jones mentioned earlier [30]. Finally, the leaders of the residency programs around the world need to establish the importance of these principles within their education systems. Programs are increasingly becoming educationally driven rather than apprentice-oriented, and part of the curriculum needs to be the principles associated with EBSP and clinical epidemiology.

References

[1] Sackett DL, Strauss SE, Richardson WS, et al. Evidence-based medicine: how to practice and teach EBM. 2nd edition. London: Churchill Livingstone; 2000.

[2] Martinez E, Pronovost P. Evidence-based anaesthesiology. In: Dawes M, Davies P, Gray A, et al, editors. Evidence-based surgery. 2000; p. 646.

[3] Dawes M. Randomized controlled trials. In: Dawes M, et al, editors. Evidence-based practice: a primer for health care professionals. London: Churchill Livingstone; 1999. p. 52.

[4] Ball CM, Phillips RS. Appendix 1: levels of evidence. In: Ball CM, Phillips RS, editors. Acute medicine. London: Churchill Livingstone; 2001. p. 641.

[5] Canadian Task Force on the Periodic Health Examination. The periodic health examination. CMAJ 1979;121:1193–254.

[6] Sackett DL. Rules of evidence and clinical recommendations on use of antithrombotic agents. Chest 1986;89(Suppl 2):2S–3S.

[7] Cook DJ, Guyatt GH, Laupacis A, et al. Clinical recommendations using levels of evidence for antithrombotic agents. Chest 1995;108(S4):227S–30S.

[8] Horton R. Surgical research or comic opera: questions, but few answers. Lancet 1996;347: 984–5.

[9] Hall JC, Hall JL. Randomisation in surgical trials. Surgery 2002;132:513–8.

[10] Howes N, Chagla L, Thorpe M, et al. Surgical practice is evidence-based. Br J Surg 1997; 84(9):1220–3.

[11] Kingston R, Barry M, Tierney S, et al. Treatment of surgical patients is evidence-based. Eur J Surg 2001;167:324–30.

[12] Wells SA Jr. Surgeons and surgical trials—why we must assume a leadership role. Surgery 2002;132:519–20.

[13] Classen DL, et al. The timing of prophylactic administration of antibiotics and the risk of surgical-wound infection. N Engl J Med 1992;326:281–6.

[14] Burke JP. Maximising appropriate antibiotic prophylaxis for surgical patients: an update from LDS Hospital, Salt Lake City. Clin Infect Dis 2001;33(Suppl 2):S78–83.

[15] Wasey N, Baughan J, de Gara CJ. Prophylaxis in elective colorectal surgery: the cost of ignoring the evidence. Can J Surg 2003;46:279–84.

[16] Bohnen JMA. Why do surgeons not comply with "best practice"? Can J Surg 2003;46.251–2.

[17] Petrowsky H, Demartines N, Rousson V, et al. Evidence-based value of prophylactic drainage in gastrointestinal surgery: a systemic review and meta-analyses. Ann Surg 2004;240: 1074–85.

[18] Nelson R, Tse B, Edwards S. Systematic review of prophylactic nasogastric decompression after abdominal operations. Br J Surg 2005;92:673–80.

[19] Dexter PR, Perkins S, Overhage JM, et al. A computerized reminder system to increase the use of preventive care for hospitalized patients. N Engl J Med 2001;345:965–70.

[20] Lenfant C. Clinical research to clinical practice—lost in translation? N Engl J Med 2003;349: 868–74.

[21] Leape L, Berwick DM. Five years after "To err is human: what have we learned?" JAMA 2005;293:2384–90.

[22] Kehlet H, Wilmore DW. Fast track surgery. In: Souba WW, Fink MP, Jurkovich OJ, et al, editors. ACS surgery. Available at: www.acssurgery.com. Accessed August 19, 2005.

[23] Basse L, Hjort Jakobse D, Billesbolle P, et al. A clinical pathway to accelerate recovery after colonic resection. Ann Surg 2000;232:51–7.

[24] Greene PS, Baumgartner WA. Cardiac surgery. In: Gordon T, Cameron JL, editors. Evidence-based surgery. Decker BC, Hamilton, Canada. 2000.

[25] Nugent WC, Schults WC. Playing by the numbers: how collecting outcomes data changed my life. Ann Thorac Surg 1994;58(6):1866–70.

[26] O'Connor GT, Plume SK, Olmstead EM, et al. A regional intervention to improve the hospital mortality associated with coronary artery bypass graft surgery. The Northern New England Cardiovascular Disease Study Group. JAMA 1996;275(11):841–6.

[27] Institute of Medicine. To err is human: building a safer health system. Washington (DC): Institute of Medicine; 1999.

[28] Institute of Medicine. Crossing the quality chasm: a new health system for the 21st century. Washington (DC): Institute of Medicine; 2001.

[29] Headline, The Times of London. August 13, 2004. p. 1.

[30] Carthey J, de Leval MR, Reason JT. The human factor in cardiac surgery errors and near misses in a high technology medical domain. Ann Thorac Surg 2001;72:300–5.

[31] Jones RS. Requiem and renewal. Ann Surg 2004;240:395–404.

[32] Meakins JL. Innovation in surgery: the rules of evidence. Am J Surg 2002;183(4):399–405.

[33] Sutton DN, Wayman J, Griffen SM. Learning curve for oesophageal cancer surgery. Br J Surg 1998;85:1399–402.

[34] McCulloch P, Taylor I, Sasako M, et al. Randomized trials in surgery: problems and possible solution. BMJ 2002;324:1448–51.

[35] Lilford R, Braunholz D, Harris J, et al. Trials in surgery. Br J Surg 2004;91:6–16.

[36] Molyneux A, Kerr R, Stratton I, et al. International Subarachnoid Aneurysm Trial (ISAT) of neurosurgical clipping versus endovascular coiling in 2143 patients with ruptured intracranial aneurysms: a randomised trial. Lancet 2002;360:1267–74.

[37] Barkun JS, Barkun AN, Sampalis JS, et al. Randomized controlled trials of laparoscopic versus mini-cholecystectomy. Lancet 1992;2:1116–9.

[38] Neumayer L, Giobbie-Hurder A, Jonasson O, et al. Open mesh versus laparoscopic mesh repair of inguinal hernia. N Engl J Med 2004;350:1819–27.

ELSEVIER
SAUNDERS

SURGICAL
CLINICS OF
NORTH AMERICA

Surg Clin N Am 86 (2006) 17–39

Knowledge Management: A Core Skill for Surgeons Who Manage

Sir Muir Gray, CBE, DSc, MD, FRCP, FRCPS(Glas)

*University of Oxford, John Radcliffe Hospital, Headington,
Oxford OX3 9DU, England, UK*

Grand Canyon: a deep gorge about 44- km long formed by the Colorado River in Arizona, USA. It is 8–24 km wide, in places 1800 m deep.
—Oxford Paperback Encyclopaedia.

The gap between what we know and what we do yawns like the Grand Canyon, but it can and must be bridged.

Health care requires revolution, not reorganization; transformation, not reformation. The new paradigm for health care has been described by different authorities, with the same themes emerging; for example, the chief executive of the National Health Service in England outlined a twenty-first century paradigm in a major conference speech in 2001 (Table 1).

Not surprisingly, as health care problems in the United States and the United Kingdom converge, a similar paradigm shift has been adopted in the United States, on the basis of the critical analysis of the reasons why quality was so low and error rates were so high in the US health care system. The first report from the Institute of Medicine, called *To Err is Human*, sent shock waves through the United States, and in the second report, called *Crossing the Quality Chasm: a New Health System for the Twenty-first Century* [1], a new approach to health care was laid out, with the contrast between the old and the new in the United States set out in Table 2.

This landmark report set out six key criteria by which health care should be measured:

1. Safety
2. Effectiveness
3. Efficiency
4. Timeliness
5. Patient-centeredness
6. Equity

E-mail address: muir.gray@dphpc.ox.ac.uk

0039-6109/06/$ - see front matter. Published by Elsevier Inc.
doi:10.1016/j.suc.2005.11.004
surgical.theclinics.com

Table 1
Health care paradigms

Twentieth century paradigm	Twenty-first century paradigm
Professional control and responsibility	Shared control and responsibility
Single professions	Teams
Expertise	Accountability
Institutions	Networks
Services	Systems
Paper	Digital
Finance as key constraint	Knowledge and people as key constraint
Quantity	Quality and safety
Averages	Inequalities
Strategy	Delivery
Science	Humanity
Centered on professionals	Centered on patients

To achieve these objectives the Chasm Report said that health care would need to be knowledge-based, patient-centered, and systems-minded (Fig. 1).

The report identified obstacles to the transformation of health care, and recommended that payment policies should facilitate, and not obstruct, quality improvement; but having removed these obstacles, the authors of the report identified three changes that needed to be made to achieve the objectives:

1. Applying evidence to clinical practice and health care delivery
2. Using information technology
3. Developing the skills and capacity of the health care work force

Knowledge is central to this process of transformation. The need to make better use of knowledge by patients and clinicians is explicitly identified in five of the ten paradigm shifts in Table 1, and is implicit in the other five.

Table 2
Approaches to health care

Current	New
Care based on visits	Care based on continuous healing
Professional autonomy drives variability	Care is customized according to patients' needs and values
Professionals control care	The patient is the source of control
Information is a record	Knowledge is shared freely
Decision-making is based on experience and training	Decision-making is based on evidence
"Do no harm"—an individual responsibility	Safety is a system property
Secrecy is necessary	Transparency is necessary
Cost reduction is sought	Waste is continuously decreased
Preference is given to professional roles over the system	Cooperation among clinicians is a priority

Adapted from Berwick DM. A user's manual for the "quality chasm." Health Affairs 2002;21:80–90.

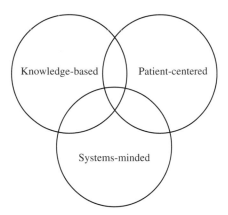

Fig. 1. Health care diagram.

Better knowledge management is necessary

The term "knowledge management" has been criticized as being misleading or banal or both, but there is a yawning gap between what we know and what we do, principally because the knowledge is not delivered to clinicians and patients where and when they need it in forms that are easy to use.

How long will it take for this knowledge to be put into practice—months, years, or never? All too often, a gap as wide as the Grand Canyon yawns between what we know and what we do, and the aim of knowledge management is to bridge that gap. To do this requires knowledge to be organized, mobilized, localized, and personalized (Fig. 2).

Three types of generalizable knowledge

"Knowledge: the sum of what is known" —Shorter Oxford English
Dictionary, 1534

There are many different ways of defining and categorizing knowledge. The author uses a simple classification based on the source of the knowledge, which may be derived from data, or research, or experience.

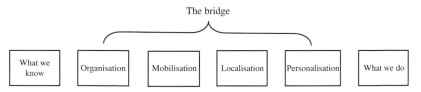

Fig. 2. Knowledge management diagram.

Knowledge derived from routinely collected or audit data

Florence Nightingale would have been the lady with the laptop, rather than the lady with the lamp, had she lived at the end of the twentieth century. Although credited with inventing nursing as a profession, her major contribution to the evolution of health care was probably to promote the use of data as a means of measuring, and then improving, quality. The use of data to improve the public health also started in the nineteenth century, when the need to tackle the great epidemics that were sweeping urbanizing Britain was recognized, but the problems of hospitals were largely ignored until Nightingale started work in the Crimea. She collected data, analyzed it, and turned it into knowledge, and with this knowledge revolutionized hospital care, first in the military hospitals and then in all hospitals.

The data derived from the performance of hospitals, and later, community health services became the main source of knowledge for people making decisions about health services during the twentieth century, with the explicit and managed use of knowledge derived from research, often called evidence, appearing only in the last decade of that century; however, although the use of data derived from performance has a long tradition, there are many controversies and uncertainties about knowledge derived from the measurement of performance.

Choosing criteria and developing systems

The data that Florence Nightingale chose to measure were strikingly obvious, namely mortality of the soldiers in the filthy hospitals of Crimea; however, she did not only measure outcome, she measured a number of different aspects of the hospital service, including the resources used, a practice that continues to this day. The terminology used to describe these sources of data varies from one country to another, but two sets of terms are commonly used: inputs and outputs, and structure and process of outcome.

Inputs and outputs are terms derived from economics: inputs are the resources put into the service (eg, numbers of doctors and nurses); outputs are the number of units work done (eg, numbers of operations or hospital admissions and discharges).

These terms were popularized by Avedis Donabedian [2], who did so much to develop thinking about the measurement of health care performance and quality assurance. The way he used the terms relate to, but are different from, inputs and outputs, namely

- Structure—the resources available, such as the number of beds or linear accelerators, analogous to the inputs of the inputs/outputs terminology
- Process—the number of treatments or episodes of care, analogous to the outputs of the inputs/outputs terminology

- Outcomes—a term used to describe the results of treatment, for example, survival following admission to intensive care or restoration of health following a coronary artery bypass grafting operation

A general term used for all of these terms is "criteria," with the concept of criteria relating to the concept of a health care system in which a system is a set of activities with a common set of objectives. For each objective, for example any screening program or hospital service, a criterion, or a number of criteria, can be chosen to allow progress toward the objectives, or lack of it, to be measured. Standards can be set, and the performance of an individual professional or service can be compared with the standard. Then, based on standards, targets can be set so that the professional or health service clearly understands the improvement in performance that is required. An example of the use of these terms in practice is set out in Table 3 [3].

In choosing criteria by which progress toward an objective can be measured, a number of criteria that can be used to measure how good the health care criteria are can be identified, and two are in common use, namely validity and feasibility.

The validity of a criterion is the degree to which it actually measures what it is intended to measure; for example, the number of complaints is a measure of patient satisfaction, but it is less valid than a systematic survey of all patients conducted by an interviewer. The feasibility of a criterion is the ease with which it can be measured. Fig. 3 sets out the relationship between these two types of criteria.

The most common type of health service criterion is the process measure, such as the number of hip replacement operations performed. Unfortunately, although hip replacement is an operation that usually produces good results, some types of artificial hip and some surgeons do not produce

Table 3
Health care standards

Objectives	Criterion	Standards		Present position	Targets
		Minimal acceptable	Achievable		
To cover the population that would benefit from cervical screening	Percentage of women who have not had a hysterectomy who have had a readable smear in the last 5 years	50%	80%	70 general practices under minimal acceptable standard; 17 practices over achievable standard	By end of the year: 1 out of 70 general practices under minimal acceptable standard; 35 general practices over achievable standard

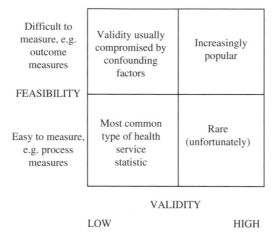

Fig. 3. Health care criteria.

such good results. There is, however, no easy way of measuring the safety and durability of a particular type of implant, or the skill of an individual surgeon, by studying the performance of one surgeon. To do this, a register has to be set up to gather sufficient information to allow valid conclusions to be drawn about a new implant or a particular surgeon, and such registers are expensive to set up and maintain, partly because they have to be maintained for many years before they can be useful.

Even when apparently useful criteria can be easily measured—such as the mortality of patients receiving treatment in a particular hospital or from a single clinician—it cannot be assumed that the criterion gives a valid measure of performance because there may be other, what are called confounding, factors. For example, the hospital or physician who is willing to treat the most advanced and difficult cases might well have a higher mortality rate than the hospital or clinician who prefers to treat only simple cases.

Comparative and public knowledge about performance

Throughout the twentieth century, hospitals, and some clinicians, kept detailed information about their performance and used this knowledge to change and improve. What we have seen in the twenty-first century, however, has been the production of comparative and public information about how one hospital compares with others and, when feasible, how the performance of one surgeon compares with others.

This process started in America when the *New York Times* took out an injunction against the New York State Health Commissioner to force the publication of mortality rates from cardiac surgery, which were eventually carried on the *New York Times* front page. The effect of this was difficult to evaluate, but it does seem that some of the surgeons who had the worst performance, principally because they were doing the fewest operations, stopped operating. In the United Kingdom the most widely publicized episode of this sort was *The Times Hospital Consultants Guide*. In the third week of November 2001, for example, *The Times of London* published five supplements, in partnership with PPP Health care, a private health care company, and Dr. Foster, a private company specializing in identifying health care information and making it available to the public. Some of these guides gave mortality rates, by hospital and not by individual clinician, and the guides gave appropriate cautionary advice about the interpretation of the death rates. For some conditions, the *Consultants Guide* concentrated on giving people information about the volume of surgery performed in different hospitals in an article explaining that "quantity is a rough guide to quality." In coronary angioplasty, for example, all the hospitals were classified as performing either 200 or more procedures per year, 20 or more procedures per year, or exceptionally or never performing these procedures.

Where death rates were provided, the paper carried good articles about the possibility that the hospitals with the higher death rates might be those treating patients with more severe or advanced disease.

The star system developed by the Commission for Health Improvement is an example of an overall indicator of a hospital's performance.

Measures or indicators

Because most criteria cannot be assumed to be perfectly valid measures of quality, some caution is always necessary when looking at hospitals or clinicians at the top or bottom of a league table, or even those that are below average, because by definition, about a half of health services will always be below average. In its report on stroke care, *The Times of London*, when reporting on 200 hospitals, wisely showed ten "above average" and ten "below average," with all the remainder in the middle, and in addition they emphasized the need to exercise judgment.

One way to think about the knowledge that we derive from performance is to regard the finding as an indicator and not a measure, just like the light on the car dashboard which, when it shines red, suggests that some action may be necessary and alerts the observer to the need to think about action, without specifying in detail what is wrong with the system.

Knowledge from research

What should we think about a doctor who uses the wrong treatment, either wilfully or through ignorance, or who uses the right treatment wrongly (such as by giving the wrong dose of a drug)? Most people would agree that such behavior was unprofessional, arguably unethical, and certainly unacceptable.

What, then, should we think about researchers who use the wrong techniques (either willfully or in ignorance), use the right techniques wrongly, misinterpret their results, report their results selectively, cite the literature selectively, and draw unjustified conclusions? We should be appalled. Yet numerous studies of the medical literature, in both general and specialist journals, have shown that all of the above phenomena are common. This is surely a scandal.

When I tell friends outside medicine that many papers published in medical journals are misleading because of methodological weaknesses they are rightly shocked [4].

The second fifty years of the twentieth century saw an astonishing increase in the number of biomedical journals, reflecting the growth in medical research and the production of evidence. The twentieth-century evidence paradigm can be summarized in a set of propositions:

- The randomized controlled trial is the definitive method for assessing effectiveness.
- The process of peer review can be relied upon to detect errors due to chance or bias, both in research applications and in articles submitted for publication.
- The main weakness of published research is the statistical methods used.
- Editorials by experts provide best current knowledge for busy clinicians.
- Textbooks provide the best source of information on treatment for students.
- Quantitative research is always better than qualitative research.
- Research is of importance to future generations of patients.

In the last decade of the twentieth century, principally because of the activities of the Cochrane Collaboration, each of these propositions came under attack, and evidence was produced to support these attacks:

- The randomized controlled trial is potentially unbiased, but in practice it has many flaws; one study of trials showed that they exaggerated the beneficial effects of treatment by up to one third [5].
- Peer review is an unreliable means of assuring quality [6].
- The main weakness of published research is its failure to build on what is already known about the subject [7].
- Editorials and reviews are often highly biased and unreliable [8].
- Textbooks are too slow to change, and often contain knowledge that is out of date, sometimes dangerously so [9].
- Primary research is often seriously flawed, but the flaws are difficult to detect in the way that the information is presented [10].

There are many reasons for this state of affairs; perhaps the most important has been over-reliance on peer review.

Rose-tinted spectacles; the unreliability of prepublication peer review

S. H. Sternberg, in his monumental book on *Five Hundred Years of Printing* [11], emphasized that one of the major benefits of the printing press was that it offered "the possibility of editing and correcting a text which was then (at least in theory) identical in every copy: in other words, mass production preceded by critical proof-reading."

At first this checking related largely to spelling and grammar, but the twentieth century saw the development of scientific journals that published the reports of research only when they had been scrutinized not only by the editor but also by an editorial committee, increasingly often advised by a system called "peer review." Hitherto the scientist was able to publish whatever he wanted, sometimes with disastrous consequences for the author, as gainfully described by Edmund Gosse in his autobiography *Father and Son*, in which his father, a distinguished biologist at the time, made himself a laughingstock by publishing a theory of evolution that sought to combine the facts of the fossil beds with the *Book of Genesis*. Peer review and the editorial process of scientific publishing, however, is not as reliable as was previously thought; the evidence is clearly summarized in an important book on the peer review process called *Peer Review in Health Sciences* [6].

Peer review fails to detect the three errors that are common in medical research:

1. Errors due to bias
2. Errors due to chance
3. Errors due to failure to incorporate research findings into the existing body of knowledge

These errors can be identified in the editorials of journals, in peer-reviewed articles in journals, in books, and on Web sites.

There is, however, another important bias that must be mentioned that is more fundamental than a failure in the peer-review process, and that is the general tendency of all those involved in research writing and publishing to emphasize the beneficial and positive aspects of research This is called "positive publication bias," and there are five main causes. These are examined in Table 4.

The twenty-first century evidence paradigm

A twenty-first century evidence paradigm has now evolved, best described in a new set of propositions:

Table 4
Five positive biases

Bias	Cause
Submission bias	Research workers are more strongly motivated to complete and submit for publication positive results
Publication bias	Editors are more likely to publish positive studies
Methodological bias	Methodological errors such as flawed randomization produce positive biases
Abstracting bias	Abstracts emphasise positive results
Framing bias	Relative risk data produce a positive bias

From Gray JAM. Evidence-based healthcare. 2nd edition. London: Churchill Livingstone; 2002. p. 108; with permission.

- Peer review has to be supplemented by other techniques to prepare knowledge for clinicians and patients; for example, the publication of journals of secondary publication or the preparation of distilled and purified evidence.
- The principal weaknesses of published research are poor study design and the failure to review previously published research in the field adequately; sophisticated statistical methodology cannot compensate for these flaws.
- Editorials, although more readable than original articles, are too unreliable to be useful for busy clinicians whose need for knowledge is better met by the production of guidelines based on systematic reviews.
- Information about treatment effectiveness is best kept up to date electronically.
- A systematic review of the evidence, formerly called "secondary research," should always precede the collection of new data, formerly called 'primary research.'
- "Primary research" published in peer-reviewed journals is an essential building block in the construction of knowledge, but clinicians, patients, and managers need knowledge that has been subjected to more rigorous quality improvement techniques than peer review.
- Qualitative research has an important contribution to make to the evidence base.

Fortunately there are now methods for creating a new knowledge paradigm based on these propositions.

The importance of qualitative research

There has always been a false dichotomy between qualitative and quantitative research. Both quantitative and qualitative research are now regarded as being essential in providing knowledge for clinicians, patients, managers, and policy-makers. Qualitative research provides a different type of information, and very often generates hypotheses that lead to quantitative studies.

For example, quantitative research is answering questions such as "Does this treatment do more good than harm?" Qualitative research, on the other hand, is very good at answering questions such as "If this treatment is beneficial in a research setting, why does it not show the same benefit in an ordinary service setting?," or "Why have professionals and patients been slow to adopt this new technique that quantitative research has shown to be effective?"

Knowledge from experience

Some of the critics of evidence-based medicine, and there were many, objected to both the term and the concept of evidence-based medicine, because it seemed to devalue the clinician's experience. Those prominent in the promotion of evidence-based medicine had, however, set out a definition that clearly distinguished between the contribution of evidence and the contribution of experience, emphasizing the importance of experience, particularly in helping to tailor evidence to the needs of the individual patient.

> Evidence-based medicine is the conscientious, explicit, and judicious use of current best evidence in making decisions about the care of individual patients. The practice of evidence-based medicine means integrating individual clinical expertise with the best available external clinical evidence from systematic research. By individual clinical expertise we mean the proficiency and judgement that individual clinicians acquire through clinical experience and clinical practice [12].

It is now recognized that knowledge from experience is of high value both for individuals and for organizations.

Learning from one's own experience: reflective practitioners

Donald Schon from Harvard wrote one of the classic books about professional practice, *The Reflective Practitioner* [13]. Studying a wide range of different professions, he developed the concept of reflective practice, as shown in the cyclical diagram in Fig. 4.

Schon pointed out that if this type of reflective learning could be enabled, it would complement the traditional training of professionals and encourage learning on the job. As part of this work, he also distinguished between the type of technical decision-making that the simple application of evidence epitomizes, and the more complicated sort of decision-making that takes into account not only the technical rationality of the scientist but also reflection based on their experience. These two examples are shown in Figs. 5 and 6.

This was a general theory applied to all professions but it can be related to medicine, as shown in Fig. 7.

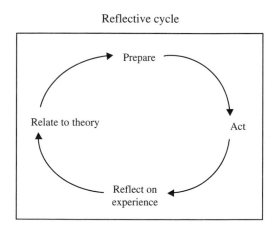

Fig. 4. Reflective practice diagram.

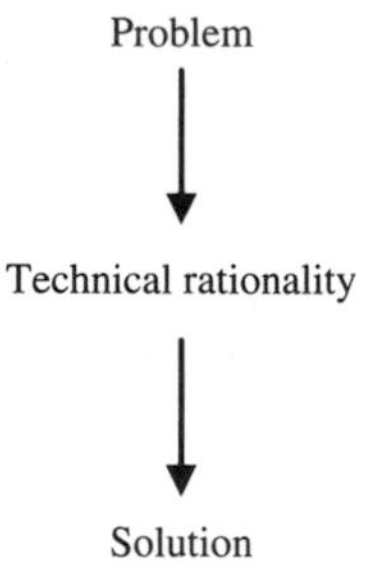

Problem

↓

Technical rationality

↓

Solution

Fig. 5. Simple decision-making diagram.

The whole principle of professional appraisal, which includes a strong element of reflection, is based on Schon's simple but elegant theory.

Learning from the experience of others

Other techniques have developed to allow teams to learn from experience.

This technique of the "after action review" was developed by the United States Army as a method of learning from experience when a team encountered an uncommon or unique situation that they, or some other team, might encounter again. One of the outputs of this process is a written document, and it is important to note that all of these systems for learning from experience require the learning to be written down, both so that it can be shared with others and as a means of making the knowledge that is inside the professional, called by some "tacit" and by others "implicit," explicit and therefore able to be shared.

The after action review relates to uncommon problems, but reflective learning can also take place when a service is offered or a process performed

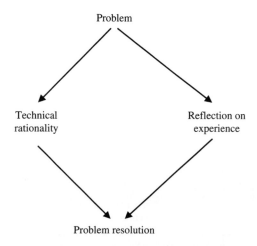

Fig. 6. Complicated decision-making diagram.

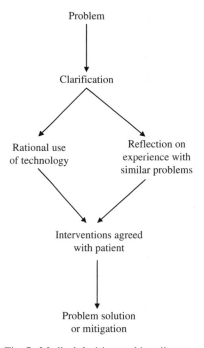

Fig. 7. Medical decision-making diagram.

continuously. The name given to such a technique is "continuous quality improvement," which may, however, go by a number of names (for example, the Japanese call it "total quality control"). It consists of a cycle analogous to Schon's cycle of reflective learning (Fig. 8).

One of the principles of continuous quality improvement is the resetting of standards, and the Japanese say that if standards are not reset annually, it

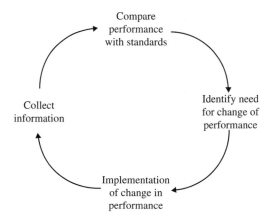

Fig. 8. Performance and quality improvement cycle.

is proof that they are not being used. The elaboration of the cycle to take into account the resetting of standards is shown in Fig. 9.

Guidelines are a way of expressing knowledge based in part on knowledge derived from research, if the guidelines claim to be evidence-based; and partly on experience, because experienced professionals have to judge how relevant the findings of a study performed in the artificial environment of research or in another country are to everyday clinical practice.

Knowledge derived from patient experience

Patients have had a great influence on clinicians; the *British Medical Journal* carries a series of accounts from doctors of patients who have changed their practices and sometimes their lives. The impact of patients has been sporadic and personal, however, and it is only in the last 10 years that a more systematic approach has been taken to the acquisition of knowledge derived from the experience of patients, and its incorporation into decision-making. In the 1980s, attention was paid to patient satisfaction, but satisfaction, although important, is not particularly helpful, because it is a function not only of the quality of service provided, but also of the patient's expectations. If expectation is low, as is commonly the case with older patients, then the patient may be grateful for a poor quality service. It is important to try to ensure that patients are satisfied, but the clinician or service manager needs knowledge that is free from the bias that expectations can impart.

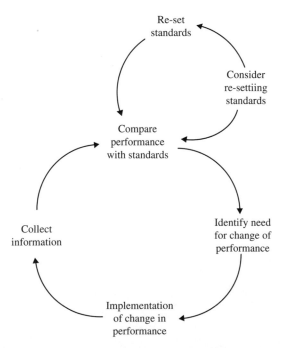

Fig. 9. Performance and quality improvement cycle, including resetting of standards.

Because of the weakness of patient satisfaction as a measure of service quality, important though it is, the Picker Institute, founded in the United States and now active in Europe, developed systematic methods for measuring the patients' experience of the care they received [14]. The Picker survey asks questions not only about the hospital environment, but also about communication and clinical decision making . Examples are listed in Box 1.

For example, rather than asking people if they were satisfied with the amount of information given, they were asked to recollect what information had been given. If the patient could not recollect any information, that fact is important to the health care organization, whether or not the clinician thought that the information had been transmitted, and whether or not the patient was satisfied with the amount of information received. The measurement of the experience provides a direct measure of service quality, and patients are resources of great value to those who provide or pay for health care.

A different type of knowledge is obtained by recording interviews with individual patients [15]. The Database of Individual Patient Experiences (DIPEX) obtained ethical approval for open interviews with patients, and for a system of editing that allowed the patient to control what went on the Web. Patients, however, are remarkably open about the information they are willing to share if they believe it will help others, and the information obtained from patients is made available as a video clip, as an audio clip, and as written text.

This type of knowledge can give useful insights to the clinician or service manager, but is of immense importance to individual patients and to professionals in training, who may not have the opportunity to hear patients who can articulate the experience of illness in the way that those who volunteer to communicate their experience to DIPEX are able to do.

Integrating the three types of knowledge

The three types of knowledge described in the previous sections are not so clearly distinguishably in practice as in theory. It might be better to consider

---

Box 1. Examples of questions on the Picker Institute Patient Survey

G3. Beforehand did a member of staff explain the risks and benefits of the operation or procedure in a way you could understand?

G4. Beforehand did a member of staff answer your questions about the operation or procedure in a way you could understand?

H5. Did a doctor explain the purpose of the medicines you were to take at home in a way you could understand?

them in the form of a Venn diagram with overlapping domains, because, for example, experience is needed to derive knowledge from research findings, and the distinction between health service statistics and research is not absolutely clear-cut.

The distinction between the three types of knowledge is, however, of some use, and the relationship between the three can be demonstrated in two ways.

One way is to show the relative importance of the three types of knowledge to clinicians, patients and managers, as shown in Fig. 10, which illustrates the knowledge matrix.

Organizing and mobilizing knowledge

It is easy to blame the individual for not being better organized, but the principal responsibility rests with the producer of knowledge. The Internet has in some ways made things easier, allowing the documents produced by an organization to be indexed and filed, updated, and retrieved, but people are now as overwhelmed by Web sites as they were once overwhelmed by paper. Each Web site becomes a knowledge silo, full of good stuff but isolated from other knowledge silos that the busy professional also needs to access. Knowledge has to be organized to meet the needs of the user, and this requires agreement on common standards for the management of documents and Web sites.

A document is, in the words of Alan Reanor, formerly Director of the Knowledge Research Centre at Brown University in Providence, Rhode Island, a "representation of knowledge objects." Most people think of documents as texts such as books and articles, but this broader definition of a document includes videos, ECG readings, patient records, audio clips, minutes of meetings, survey forms, and other sources of information as well.

When knowledge is properly organized, it can then mobilized, and anyone who wishes to mobilize knowledge has to think not only of pull, but also of push and prompt (Fig. 11).

	Knowledge from research	Knowledge from experience	Knowledge from data
Patient	✓	✓	✓
Clinician	✓✓	✓✓	✓
Managers	✓	✓	✓✓

Fig. 10. Knowledge matrix. ✓, less relevant; ✓✓, more relevant.

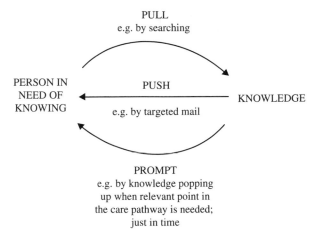

Fig. 11. Just-in-time knowledge: pull, push, and prompt.

Push: delivering urgent knowledge

If a fault is found in an orange wire in a particular type of aircraft engine, every mechanic in the world responsible for checking the engine will know within hours to check that orange wire; in the health service, safety notices may take days or months or years to reach the person who needs to know, sometimes too late to prevent harm. Some knowledge is not only important, it is also urgent, and it must be delivered to the clinicians and patients who need to know within a day of its becoming available so that action can be taken.

This requires, first, a system for identifying the knowledge that is both important and urgent, because it is even more important from an ethical perspective to deliver knowledge about potential harm than to deliver knowledge about the potential benefits of a drug or treatment. Of equal importance is the presence of a system for delivering urgent knowledge, and although there are cascade systems for health care professionals that work well for major problems, the development of e-mail allows urgent knowledge to be pushed at relatively small groups of professionals, for example, all neurologists.

Every organization that produces knowledge needs to have a marketing strategy, with the key customers for their knowledge projects clearly identified. The blunderbuss approach of sending knowledge to everyone may mean that those who most need to know do not see it, and the circulation list of a paper about the prevention of rhesus iso-immunization disease illustrates the scale of the problem if it is not possible to target those people who must urgently need to know.

When Ford is launching a new model, it produces 6000 pages of documentation, both digital and paper, in 23 languages, targeted at different groups of individuals whose names and locations are known, and in the expectation that at least 20 updates will be needed in the first year.

If Ford can do this for its communities of practice, for its salesmen and mechanics, surely a health service can do the same for clinicians and patients.

Prompt: delivering just-in-time knowledge

Storage consumes resources. As part of the industrial revolution called "lean thinking," the delivery of the components that the car production line needed was streamlined so that the components arrived just in time, delivered straight from the producer to the worker on the production line, doing away with the need for warehouses, inventories, storage facilities, shelving, and all the paraphernalia required when supplies are unnecessarily stored. As with a car production line, so with a clinical care pathway. Instead of the clinician having to leave the care pathway and ferret about in the knowledge stores to find the knowledge that is needed, it is simpler to deliver the knowledge to the clinician, and to the patient, during the process of care. The knowledge can be delivered just in time in the way that car components are delivered just in time when the production worker on the Toyota assembly line has need of a windshield or windshield wiper.

Providing the opportunity of searching during the consultation or on the ward round allows the clinician to mobilize knowledge, and improved access to knowledge will make a big difference, as a famous study of the use of the evidence cart in Oxford's John Radcliffe Hospital demonstrated [16]. By having the ability to search on the ward round, the A team at the John Radcliffe asked more questions and found more answers, many of which had a significant impact on patient care. They did this because of the ease of searching, and the team found that in the time taken to walk to and from the library they could carry out 16 searches. Of the searches completed on the ward, 52% confirmed the current diagnosis, 25% led to a change in care, and 23% corrected a test or treatment.

When the facility was removed, the team continued to identify the need for evidence, but only searched for it in 12% of the times that evidence was needed, because of the barriers to searching that a walk from the ward to the library entailed. The team showed that when knowledge was available, more questions were asked; but the provision of knowledge just in time does not need to rely on the clinician asking the question—the clinician can be prompted to ask the appropriate question.

The worker on the Toyota production line reaches for a windshield not because he has suddenly asked a question, "What do I need next?," but because an embryonic car is moving toward him with a space where the windshield should be, and the worker is prompted to reach for the windshield. The development of digital care pathways allows the opportunity for clinicians to be prompted with information they might need. For example, a digital care pathway allows the clinician to be offered prompts and reminders about, for example

Indications for referral
Drug side effects
Patient information leaflets that can be printed off immediately
Current randomized controlled trials that the patient might wish to enter

Localization

Knowledge from research is generalizable and valid in countries other than those in which the research was performed; however, the research findings cannot necessarily be assumed to be applicable in every country, because there might be differences in the resources available or the organization and funding of health services. Knowledge from research, therefore, has to be combined with knowledge from experience when a national guideline is being produced (Fig. 12).

National guidelines are often monumental documents, and may be 200 or more pages long. To be useful, national guidelines have to be localized; that is, made relevant to a particular service as what are called "protocols." Protocols allow guidelines to be modified to take into account constraints in a particular service; for example, a deficiency in that service that would be required to implement the guideline fully. In addition, localization can include information of relevance only to patients and clinicians in a particular service; for example, key telephone numbers and local contacts, so that a single document helps the clinician get the knowledge into action (Fig. 13).

The local protocol is usually shorter than the national guideline, but it still has to be consulted separately from the clinical episode, so the next

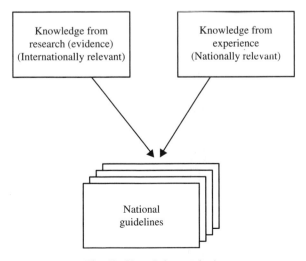

Fig. 12. Knowledge synthesis.

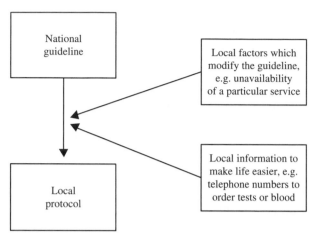

Fig. 13. Generating local protocols from national guidelines.

stage in localization is to create a care pathway; for example, the care pathway for a chest pain clinic or for a patient needing knee replacement surgery. The care pathway is a form incorporating decision support from a local protocol and useful local information. The care pathway for knee replacement surgery, for example, might include the need to provide the patient with elastic stockings (knowledge generated from research), and the need to cross-match blood, with the telephone number and the details of how to send a sample in to the hematology laboratory (knowledge from experience).

Where a pathway is made available as part of the electronic patient record, it is sometimes called a digital care pathway.

Localization can, however, serve another function than tailoring the national guideline to local circumstances; it can also increase the emotional commitment of clinicians to a nationally produced document, a form of personalization.

Personalization

The first type of cake mix was made by Mary Baker, who discovered that a powdered cake mix only became acceptable to the American housewife when she took out the powdered egg and required the woman, for men did not make cakes in the 1950s, to break in a real egg; the same process is required for guideline adoption. National guidelines have a strong evidence base but low acceptability. Locally produced guidelines, as opposed to local protocols based on national guidelines, were high in acceptability but often low on the strength of the evidence on which the guideline was based (Fig. 14).

The development of local protocols from national guidelines ensures both a strong evidence base and acceptability.

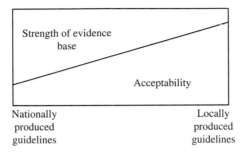

Fig. 14. National versus local guidelines: strength and acceptability.

There is, however, a second stage in personalization that the clinician has to undertake. Although knowledge is generalizable from one country to another when applied to groups of patients, the act of relating knowledge to the individual patient is a second form of personalization that clinicians have to perform. The clinician acts like a tailor, measuring and cutting the evidence to match the patient's particular circumstances and values.

Using knowledge

Even if all these steps are taken, the knowledge still has to be put into practice, and that requires individuals, both patients and clinicians, who are hungry for knowledge and know how to use it, and organizations that facilitate the use of knowledge in decision-making. This is one of the benefits from the introduction of evidence-based surgery.

Allocating responsibility for knowledge management

Every health care organization should have a chief knowledge officer, someone on the management board who is responsible for ensuring that the organization imports the knowledge it needs, that there are systems in place that move the knowledge to those who need it, and that any publications, reports and patient leaflets produced by the organization are evidence-based and quality-assured.

Every hospital needs a chief knowledge officer, but so too does every division of surgery. Intellectual resources need to be managed as carefully as financial or human resources. This structural change is, however, only one change that organizations need to make. Organizations also have systems and a culture, and these three are inter-related (Fig. 15).

A division of surgery needs systems for

- Scanning new evidence
- Identifying dilemmas of either individual clinical care or management for which evidence is unclear, and attempting to clarify the evidence

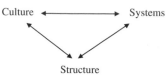

Fig. 15. Components of organizations.

- Ensuring that newly recruited members of staff are aware of the evidence base on which the Division operates
- Doing research or facilitating the research of others, including the preparation of systematic reviews
- Purchasing equipment using evidence as well as price; the cheapest equipment is not necessarily the best.

The responsibility for doing this can rest with the chairman of the division, or be allocated to another surgeon, and that person will need the support of a well-trained librarian.

The knowing–doing gap

The yawning gap between what we know and what we do has major implications for patients and populations. By putting into practice what we know at present, we will have a bigger impact on the health of individuals and populations than any drug or new technology likely to be discovered in the new decade will have. The assumption underlying this article is that the gap can be bridged, and that the gap between what we know and what we do can be closed by taking thought, planning, analyzing, mobilizing, managing, personalizing, and using knowledge. It is reasonable to

---

Box 2. Why typical knowledge management practices made knowing-doing gaps worse

- Knowledge management efforts mostly emphasize technology and the transfer of codified information.
- Knowledge management tends to treat knowledge as a tangible thing, as a stock or a quantity, and therefore separates knowledge as some *thing* from the use of that thing.
- Formal systems can't easily store or transfer tacit knowledge.
- The people responsible for transferring and implementing knowledge management frequently don't understand the actual work being documented.
- Knowledge management tends to focus on specific practices and ignore the importance of philosophy.

assume that this hypothesis is correct. There is, however, a danger that the attempted solution may perpetuate or aggravate the problem, and a powerful book called *The Knowing-Doing Gap: How Smart Companies turn Knowledge into Action* [17] describes the dangers of substituting thought for action. In the chapter called "Knowing What to Do Is Not Enough," the authors include a list of management practices that make the knowing-doing gap worse, presented in Box 2.

The danger described here can develop when knowledge management becomes an industry with a life of its own, remote from the core activities of the organization and from those who deliver them. The authors also include a very useful checklist that the perceptive professional can use to spot when the process of mobilizing knowledge and planning actually slows down action.

References

[1] Institute of Medicine. Crossing the quality chasm: a new health system for the twenty-first century. Washington, DC: National Academy Press; 2001.

[2] Donabedian A. The definition of quality: a conceptual exploration. In: Explorations in quality assessment and monitoring. Volume I: The definition of quality and its approaches to its assessment. Ann Arbor (MI): Health Administration Press; 1980.

[3] Gray JAM. Evidence-based healthcare. 2nd edition. London: Churchill Livingstone; 2002.

[4] Altman D. The scandal of poor medical research. BMJ 1994;308:283–4.

[5] Schulz KF, Chalmers I, Haynes RJ, et al. Empirical evidence of bias: dimensions of methodological quality associated with estimates of treatment effects in controlled trials. JAMA 1995;273:408–12.

[6] Jefferson T, Godlee F. Peer review in health sciences. London: BMJ Publications; 1999.

[7] Chalmers I, Clarke M. Discussion sections in reports of controlled trials published in general medical journals: islands in search of continents. JAMA 1998;280:280–2.

[8] Mulrow CW. The medical review article: state of the science. Ann Intern Med 1987;106: 485–8.

[9] Antman EM, Lau J, Kupelnick B, et al. A comparison of results of meta-analysis of randomized control trials and recommendations of clinical experts. JAMA 1992;268:240–8.

[10] Chalmers TC, Frank CS, Reitman D. Minimizing the three stages of publication bias. JAMA 1990;263:1392–5.

[11] Sternberg SH. Five hundred years of printing. London: The British Library; 1996.

[12] Sackett DL, Rosenberg WM, Gray JAM, et al. Evidence based medicine: what it is and what it isn't. BMJ 1996;312:71–2.

[13] Schon DA. The reflective practitioner. New York: Basic Books; 1991.

[14] Available at: http://www.pickereurope.org. Accessed December 24, 2005.

[15] Available at: http://www.dipex.org.uk. Accessed December 24, 2005.

[16] Sackett DL, Straus SE. The evidence cart. Finding and applying evidence during the clinical round. JAMA 1998;280:1336–8.

[17] Pfeffer J, Sutton R. Knowing doing gap. Boston; 1999.

SURGICAL
CLINICS OF
NORTH AMERICA

Surg Clin N Am 86 (2006) 41–57

Finding and Appraising Evidence

Peter McCulloch, MD, FRCSEd[a,*],
Douglas Badenoch, MSc[b]

[a]Nuffield Department of Surgery, Oxford University, Level 6, John Radcliffe Hospital,
Headington, Oxford OX3 9DU, United Kingdom
[b]Minervation Ltd 7200 The Quorum, Oxford Business Park North, Oxford,
OX4 2JZ, United Kingdom

Surgeons have tended to regard evidence-based medicine with a degree of skepticism. A variety of reasons for this have been proposed, ranging from the surgical personality to the nature of the research questions that occur when studying surgical treatment. The relative paucity of randomized trials of surgical treatment has been noted by many investigators [1], and there has been considerable debate about whether this reflects poorly on the scientific education of the surgical community or points to special problems in applying this methodology in this discipline.

This debate has matured over the last 10 years, and there is now on the one hand greater understanding of the special factors that make surgical operations difficult subjects for randomized trials [2]; on the other hand, such trials are being done now more than ever before.

The importance of this uneasy history of the surgeon searching for evidence to support clinical decisions is clear. The amount of randomized trial evidence is likely to be small in many areas. This does mean that finding and appraising the most reliable evidence on a given subject is not likely to take long, but the plethora of information about studies (mainly case series) with poorer designs often tends to overshadow the limited trial evidence, especially where the conclusions of the two conflict. In this regard, surgery is in the same boat as a number of other specialities such as public health, where many questions cannot be definitively answered from the results of randomized trials.

Nevertheless, we are where we are. Being able to extract the most relevant studies from the literature is still a crucial skill for the modern surgeon, for a number of reasons. First, if there really is no valid evidence about a subject,

* Corresponding author.
E-mail address: peter.mcculloch@nds.ox.ac.uk (P. McCulloch).

this may be important. Many surgical conventions, such as the use of naso-gastric tubes and drains, are governed far more by tradition and apprentice-ship than by evidence; if we can be confident that there is no evidence to support them, we are more likely to challenge them. No subject can advance by always doing what our predecessors did, so such challenges are likely, if they lead to appropriately designed trials, to improve the overall quality of treatment.

Second, analysis of nontrial evidence using the principles of evidence-based medicine, and particularly a clear understanding of the likelihood and sources of bias, will leave us in a better position to state the limits of our ignorance. Case series cannot generally prove one treatment superior to another, but they can provide convincing evidence that a treatment is of-ten followed by a satisfactory outcome. If there is good evidence about the natural history of the untreated condition (eg, malignant large bowel ob-struction), this can be powerful evidence that the intervention is of value, even though factors such as the balance with potential harm and the effects of selection bias need to be carefully considered.

Finally, the disparate nature of the surgical literature means that we are often surprised at what we find. There may indeed be randomized trial ev-idence on the question we are interested in, even if we have never before been aware of it. One of the authors was recently surprised to find out that there were at least 13 randomized trials on gastric reservoir procedures after total gastrectomy, an area of specialized expertise in which said author was confident that the literature was almost entirely anecdotal. As with most other areas of health care, there is no lack of information, and there are many different searchable databases.

Finding the best evidence

This section discusses the basic principles of searching for evidence and suggests some pointers for making the best use of limited searching time. Some useful tips include (Fig. 1):

AND: Retrieve documents which match BOTH of the conditions you specify
a AND b

OR: Retrieve documents which match EITHER of the conditions you specify
a OR b

NOT: Retrieve documents which match the first condition you specify BUT NOT the second.
a NOT b

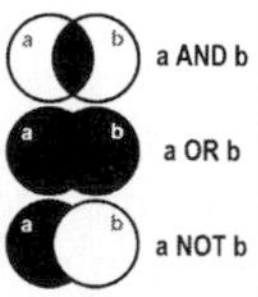

Proximity Operators:
ADJ: Terms must appear next to each other
NEXT: As above
NEAR: Terms must appear within a certain number of words from each other

Fig. 1. Boolean operators.

Use the PICO (Patient, Intervention, Comparison, Outcome) format to structure your search.

By beginning with the PICO format, you can make sure that your search query is specific. This simple rephrasing of the clinical question in a standard structure helps to clarify exactly what should be included and excluded from your search. This gives you the best chance of finding a manageable number of relevant hits.

Prioritize the questions that matter most to your practice.

You probably have little time to do systematic searching, so choose the topics that are most likely to make a difference in your practice.

Start with secondary sources.

Systematic reviews and evidence-based journals contain information that has already been appraised by people who (hopefully) know what they're doing, so they can give you a shortcut to the answer you need.

In primary sources, use filters to weed out the dross at source.

Most databases can be limited by publication type, and many have "filters" that can target the higher-quality study designs according to your question type. Your local librarian can help you do this if there is no filter available [3].

Use a thesaurus.

The documents coded into a database are usually assigned index terms to describe what they are about. You can browse (or search) these terms in a thesaurus to find all of the documents relating to that term. This is a good way to conduct a specific search, though you may miss some items.

Asking answerable questions

The most common mistake when searching for evidence is to type one concept (such as "radical prostatectomy") into a database and be overwhelmed by thousands of hits. We are then at the mercy of the database's choice of what to put at the top of the list. The best way around this is to make sure that you have a clear definition of the question you want answered.

In clinical practice, clearly focused questions usually have four components: patient, intervention, comparison, and outcome, otherwise known as the PICO format (Table 1) [4]. The PICO format is useful because [5]:

- it is easier to remember natural language questions
- it helps you build an effective search strategy by identifying key terms
- you can discount studies that do not address your question
- It is a useful framework for considering how applicable a study would be in your context

Prioritizing your questions

Studies suggest that there can be as many as three questions for every patient encounter [6]. Clearly, we cannot rush off to the library every time, so we need to prioritize the ones that matter most.

Table 1
Question components

Component	Description	Example
Patient	A description of your patient, including their clinical condition	A man aged 70 with nonmetastatic prostate cancer
Intervention	What you are considering doing	Radical prostatectomy
Comparison	What the alternative would be	Watchful waiting
Outcomes	The events that you are trying to prevent (or bring about)	Occurrence of metastases, overall survival time

In men aged 70 with non-metastatic prostate cancer, does radical prostatectomy, as compared with watchful waiting, prevent the spread of disease or increase survival time?

The convention in medical and surgical education is to focus on the unusual, interesting cases. This is stimulating and challenging, but most of what we learn in such exercises is forgotten immediately or is never put into practice [5]. We recommend the opposite: concentrate on questions that are likely to recur in your practice. That way you will get the best benefit from the small amount of time you have available to you. By capturing and storing the answers in the form of critically appraised topics (CATs) you can build up a specialized evidence base relevant to your own practice and share the load of finding the evidence amongst your team and colleagues [7].

It is important to consider what type of question you are asking, because that will determine what type of research you need to answer it. The main categories of question, and the best study designs for answering them, are shown in Table 2.

Table 3 provides additional details on what to look for in these types of studies. The section on searching online databases discusses how some databases allow you to filter the right type of study to fit your type question.

For all question types, however, the best type of study is one in which someone has already done all the work of finding, assessing, and summarizing the relevant evidence. Thus you should always start your search by looking for such secondary sources, because this may save much time and effort.

Table 2
Question type and study type

Question type	Study type
Diagnosis	Prospective validation study with blind, independent comparison against a gold standard of diagnosis
Etiology or harm	Case–control or cohort study
Prognosis	Cohort study
Treatment or prevention	Randomized controlled trial
Cost-effectiveness	Economic evaluation
Quality of Life	Qualitative research

Table 3
Sources of evidence

Database	Media	Vendors	Contents
Secondary sources			
Clinical evidence	Online service, books	BMJ Publishing	Treatment and harm in all aspects of medicine where good evidence already exists
Cochrane Library Systematic reviews Controlled Trials Register DARE abstracts Economic analyses	Online service, CD-ROM	Wiley, Update Software	Systematic reviews of (mostly) treatments, RCTs and cost-effectiveness analyses in all branches of medicine
ACP Journal Club	Online service, CD-ROM (best evidence), journal	ACP, Ovid (via evidence-based medicine reviews subscription)	Appraised and relevance-filtered summaries of key publications in medicine
Trip Database	Online service	www.tripdatabase.com	Appraised summaries of key publications in medicine
CAT Crawler	Online service	http://www.bii-sg.org/ research/mig/ cat_search.asp	CATCrawler searches collections of critically appraised topics on the Internet
Primary sources			
Medline	Internet, online service, CD-ROM	PubMed, Ovid, SilverPlatter, Dialog/Datastar, and other vendors	Medicine and surgery (United States focus)
EMBASE	Online service	PubMed, Ovid, SilverPlatter, Dialog/Datastar, and other vendors	Medicine and pharmacology (Europe focus)

Abbreviations: CAT, critically appraised topics; DARE, database of abstracts of reviews of effectiveness; RCTs, randomized controlled trials.

Secondary sources

You will make the most of your searching time if you look for material that summarizes or reviews primary research. This includes:

- clinical guidelines (eg, SIGN)
- health technology assessments (eg, NICE technology appraisals)
- structured abstracts (eg, ACP Journal Club)
- evidence syntheses (eg, clinical evidence)

- systematic reviews (eg, Cochrane Library) (Box 1)
- critically appraised topics (eg, BestBETs)

Good databases for such documents are shown in Table 3.

Of course, you will want to be satisfied that the process by which these summaries were created was up to snuff. Look for:

- a "purpose and procedure" section that explains how the primary research was found and appraised
- an independent review of the output
- an effective mechanism for keeping reviews up-to-date

Unfortunately, secondary sources are few and far between in surgery, so you may often have to consult primary sources for your answer. This may also be true if you decide that the summary was not of high quality or did not specifically answer your question.

Primary sources

A primary source is a document that contains the original report of a study. Tens of thousands of such papers are published every year, so it can be a daunting prospect.

Bibliographic databases contain millions of records (references) describing many different kinds of publications, usually including an abstract. When you search them, you are looking for the occurrences of your search terms in these references. Because of their size, it's important to be careful how you search these databases (Box 2, Fig. 2).

Box 1. Systematic reviews

A systematic review is a secondary publication in which the authors have systematically identified, retrieved, appraised, and synthesized all of the previous research about a clinical question into a single conclusion. In other words, systematic reviews can be the best evidence possible about a clinical question.

This might sound too good to be true, and it sometimes is. You will want to check that:

- the reviewers did not miss any important studies
- the reviewers did not include poor-quality research that might bias the results
- it makes sense to combine the individual studies into one

Sadly, you will find that many clinical questions do not yet have a systematic review.

Box 2. Text word versus thesaurus searching

There are two ways to search a bibliographic database:
(1) text word searching and (2) thesaurus searching. In text word searching, you type words into a search box and the database will find records that contain those words. In thesaurus searching, you can search or browse a subject index (such as MeSH) and retrieve documents that a human indexer has assigned to your topics.

If you wish to be comprehensive, it is important to use both techniques because: (1) the text words in a bibliographic record may not be the same ones you thought of in your text word search, so you should use the thesaurus as well; and (2) indexers can make mistakes when assigning index terms, so you cannot rely on a thesaurus search alone.

Which database?

There are hundreds of different biomedical databases (see Table 3). Choose the few that matter to you on the basis of:

- relevant subject coverage
- whether they contain secondary sources such as systematic reviews

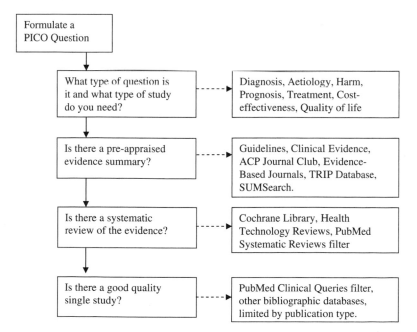

Fig. 2. Finding the evidence flow chart.

- balancing the need to be comprehensive with time available for searching

Principles of searching online databases

Although each vendor has a different method of searching, they all conform to the same basic principles.

The next step is deciding how much it matters to be comprehensive. For example, what if you miss some relevant documents? If comprehensiveness is not important, you can use a thesaurus (or index); otherwise, you will have to combine a thesaurus search with a "free text" (or textword) search (Box 3).

Stop words

Most databases ignore words such as *most*, *do*, *not*, and *like*, so there is little to be gained by searching for them.

Sample search from PubMed

Table 4 shows a sample search in which we selected the most important concepts from our PICO question and input them into PubMed. Some points of note:

Box 3. In a 70-year-old man with nonmetastatic prostate cancer, a prostate-specific antigen test score of 15, and Gleason score of 8, does radical prostatectomy, as compared with watchful waiting, increase life expectancy?

Translate your PICO question into search terms
Aged 70
Prostate cancer
Radical prostatectomy
Watchful waiting
Survival time

Build up individual terms using AND
"watchful AND waiting"

Combine equivalent terms with OR
"watch-and-wait"
"1 OR 2"
"radical ADJ prostatectomy"
"survival" OR "mortality"

Combine different parts of the PICO question using AND
"3 AND 4 AND 5"

Table 4
Sample PubMed search history

Search	Most recent queries	Time	Result
#11	Search #6 AND #7 AND #10	06:54:11	74
#10	Search #9 OR #8	06:53:36	719050
#8	Search mortality	06:53:08	460605
#9	Search survival	06:52:47	438459
#7	Search radical prostatectomy	06:52:02	6645
#6	Search #3 OR #4 OR #5	06:51:21	19672
#5	Search watch-and-wait	06:51:00	104
#4	Search active surveillance	06:50:40	18899
#3	Search watchful waiting	06:50:30	688

1. "Watchful waiting" has no MeSH heading, so we have to combine all the different ways in which this concept can be described using OR. Notice how line 6 has more hits than line 3, 4, or 5.
2. It is worth checking the *Details* tab on PubMed to see how the database translated each line of your search. For example, if you enter "survival" into the search box and click *Details*, you get:
   - "mortality" [Subheading] OR "survival" [MeSH Terms] OR survival [Text Word]

   By comparison, if you enter "mortality" into the search box, you get:
   - "mortality" [Subheading] OR "mortality" [MeSH Terms] OR mortality [Text Word]

This underlines why it is important to combine terms and not just rely on PubMed to cover all your possibilities.

3. For very specific terms, such as "radical prostatectomy", the PubMed interfaces work very well at translating it into both a textword and MeSH search:
   - radical [All Fields] AND ("prostatectomy" [MeSH Terms] OR prostatectomy [Text Word])
4. Finally, we have used OR to build up a search for each PICO concept separately; we then use AND to combine them into our question.

PubMed clinical queries

One of the best services PubMed offers is the ability to target your search using the Clinical Queries feature (http://www.ncbi.nlm.nih.gov/entrez/query/static/clinical.shtml; linked on the left hand menu on http://www.pubmed.gov).

This allows you to type in a topic, select your question type (etiology, diagnosis, therapy or prognosis) and do a search for the best type of research to answer your question.

For example, for a therapy question, PubMed will take your topic (eg, radical prostatectomy) and create a query automatically that looks for randomized controlled trials using a validated "search filter".

In this particular example, PubMed transforms your two words into the following search: (radical [All Fields] AND ("prostatectomy" [MeSH Terms] OR prostatectomy [Text Word])) AND (randomized controlled trial [Publication Type] OR (randomized [Title/Abstract] AND controlled [Title/Abstract] AND trial [Title/Abstract]))

The methods PubMed uses have been validated against a test-set of documents, so you can have confidence that they will be accurate.

PubMed is gradually adding to these services, with topic-based filters as well as methodological filters. There is a cancer filter available at http://www.ncbi.nlm.nih.gov/entrez/query.fcgi?db=PubMed&orig_db=PubMed&cmd_current=Limits&pmfilter_Subsets=Cancer.

Other MEDLINE vendors

Commercial information services, most notably Ovid and Dialog, also offer access to Medline and many other databases through one interface. Their principal advantage is that you can search many different databases at the same time; the principal disadvantage is that a paid subscription is required. Some services, notably Ovid, offer value-added databases such as "Evidence-Based Medicine Reviews."

The searching techniques we have described above are applicable to all databases. What you should look out for are:

- differences in how thesaurus and textword searching is implemented: use the Search History or Details option to see exactly how the database has searched
- variations in the use of operators and wildcards, especially the proximity operators
- how much it costs and whether you can get free access

You should consult your local library service to find out exactly what you can get and how best to use it. There may be other helpful resources, such as the ISI Web of Knowledge, which contains the Science Citation Index as well as MEDLINE; Biological Abstracts; and other biomedical databases that are not covered by MEDLINE.

A final note: most databases now allow you to set up "alert" services, in which you can have relevant material e-mailed to you as soon as it is added to the database.

Searching the Internet

Search engines

Internet search engines work by trawling the internet examining the contents of Web pages and sending information about them back to an index in a central database. It is this database you search when you type your terms into the search engine.

You then get a list of "hits" ranked according to how relevant the database thinks each item is to your query. Because of the sheer quantity of material on the net, your main challenge will be to find relevant material and reduce the number of hits you get.

Fortunately, the most popular search engines are very effective at placing more relevant hits at the top of the ranking. Exactly how they do this varies (and is shrouded in secrecy). However, most of them place a higher weight on pages that have a lot of links from other Web sites, on the assumption that if people think they're worth linking to, they're more likely to be useful. They may also give a higher weight where your search terms occur in the title of the page.

Search tips

- Use three or four of your terms at once: search engines will only retrieve documents which match all of them, so you're more likely to succeed.
- Don't use "stopwords" (see above)
- Use quotes to search for an exact phrase (eg, "radical prostatectomy")

Limitations

- Indexing site content: not all the information on the internet is indexed. Some might be "buried" in a site: if you find a large site containing lots of potentially relevant documents, it's worth doing a search using the site's own search engine to see if you can pick up any additional hits.
- Updating: you might find that some links are dead because the site has changed since it was indexed.

Specialist search engines

Google Scholar (http://scholar.google.com) searches academic papers, journal articles and similar databases on the internet. You'll find, for example, peer-reviewed articles, technical reports, PubMed citations, PDF, Word and PowerPoint presentation using this portal.

Ask Medline (http://www.ulb.ac.be/erasme/en/biblio-medline.htm) is a highly simplified interface to PubMed. Type a question into the box and it will transform your search into a PubMed query and show you the results. It is good for specific queries (not so good if you want high sensitivity) and for those who find the PubMed interface off-putting.

Deciding on quality

Critical appraisal

There are three possible explanations for the results of any study:

The study was biased toward producing that result.

The result happened by chance.
The result happened because it represents the truth.

Critical appraisal is about ruling out the first two possibilities.

Deciding on validity

There are three things you need to ask yourself about any piece of evidence you find:

Does it address a clearly focused, relevant question?
Is it valid? (Box 4)
Are the valid results important?

If the answer to any one of these questions is "No," you can save yourself the trouble of going any further.

We have already addressed the PICO question—so all that should be said is that you must be satisfied that the study defines these components clearly, and in satisfactory clinical terms before you can answer "Yes" to the first question.

How we assess validity depends on the type of question we are addressing (see Table 5). In general terms:

- prospective research is more likely to be valid than retrospective research
- outcome assessment should not be influenced by knowledge of how subjects were selected (sampling) or of what was done to whom (performance)

Where does bias come from?

There is good evidence that the results of research are affected by bias. For a good, readable review, see *The Bandolier Guide to Bias* [8]. Clinicians, especially those who have done some clinical research themselves, tend to be skeptical about the effects of bias, but often miss the point that what we are talking about is unconscious interference with the fairness of a study. Conscious interference is called fraud. The bottom line is that, in general terms, bias leads us to overestimate the effectiveness of what we do.

Box 4. Validity

Validity means different things to different people. There are
    fancy technical definitions of internal and external validity,
    construct validity, and so forth. What we mean by validity is:
    "Are the methods used likely to produce a biased result?"

Table 5
Study characteristics by question type

Question type	Selection	Performance	Ascertainment
Diagnosis	Was the test validated on an appropriate spectrum of patients?	Was the test compared with a reference standard, regardless of the experimental test result?	Were the test results ascertained by investigators who were blinded to the patient's true condition?
Prognosis	Was the sample well-defined, representative, and at a common point in disease progression?	Was follow-up long enough and complete enough?	Were outcomes assessed blind to sample or individual characteristics?
Etiology	Were the groups matched for all the clinically important factors apart from the exposure?	Was follow-up long enough and complete enough?	Were exposures and outcomes measured in the same way in both groups?
Treatment	Were the groups the same at the start of the trial (randomization and allocation concealment)?	Were the groups treated equally throughout (blinding of patients and caregivers)?	Were outcomes assessed blind to treatment?

No one likes to believe that they are wasting their time, especially when there may be millions of dollars invested in developing a new treatment. Unfortunately, this can (and has) led us to do things that are ineffective and even harmful to patients, such as prescribing the antiarrhythmic flecainide to patients after myocardial infarction [9]. Even now, in the era of evidence-based medicine, we have seen the example of Vioxx, which may have caused between 88,000 and 140,000 myocardial infarctions or sudden cardiac deaths in the United States alone [10].

What matters most in checking for bias?

Studies of bias have shown that the most common source is unfair sampling of patients, known as selection bias [11]. When comparing two different groups, you must be confident that they are similar in all important ways apart from the experimental intervention. In therapy trials, the only way to be sure of this is by randomly assigning recruits to the different treatment groups. However, randomization can still be messed up if the person who recruits patients finds out which treatment group is up next. This is known as allocation concealment.

The next most important thing is to make sure that the subjects were treated the same during the study. The only way to be sure of this is to prevent the patients, their caregivers, and the assessors of outcome (if different) knowing which group each patient is in. This can be relatively easy (eg, a placebo tablet in a drug trial) or very challenging (eg, concealing which of two operative procedures has been done).

Sample checklist for therapy study

Was treatment group assigned randomly? If so, was the randomization
list concealed? (Concealing the list is done to prevent peeking in the en-
velope and similar cheating, which may seem trivial but may increase
the estimated treatment effect by as much as 30%.)

Were the randomly selected groups similar at the start of the trial?

Were the experimental and control groups treated in the same way apart
from the allocated therapy?

Were all patients who started the trial accounted for at the end? If so,
were their outcomes analyzed by "intention to treat"? That is, were
they counted in the group they were allocated to, even if they did
not receive the treatment intended? This can be important, for example, for effective treatments with bad side effects, in which case only
a minority of allocated patients can complete the course. Analyzing
the results of only the ones who did complete the course would give
a false impression of the usefulness of the treatment.

Were there clear measures of outcome?

Were patients and observers kept blind as to the treatment given? (This is
difficult in many surgical studies but is not impossible.)

Was the follow-up long enough?

The bottom line is that if we do not look for bias in clinical research, we
risk harming our patients.

Sample size

It is important to determine if there were enough patients in a study to
show a significant finding. There are complicated statistical methods for
determining the right sample size. They depend on four factors, which the
researchers must determine beforehand:

The baseline risk of the outcome (rare outcomes require more patients).

The expected benefit (how much improvement the researchers want to be
able to detect).

The type 1 error risk (the risk of falsely believing the finding to be significant when it isn't; this is called *alpha*, and the acceptable risk of type 1
error is conventionally set at 5%).

The type 2 error risk (the risk of falsely believing the finding to be non-
significant when it is, or *beta*, which is conventionally set at 20%).
Note: $1 - \beta =$ is sometimes known as the *significance level* and may
be expressed as "The study was powered to have an 80% chance of
detecting a 10% relative risk reduction."

Thankfully, you need not worry about the ins and outs of calculating
sample size: if the study did not have enough patients in it, you will be
able to tell from the confidence interval around the results.

Confidence intervals

Every study requires that a sample be taken from a population. The chances are that the sample will differ from the population in some ways; thus, the results may be different from the true value of the population.

Confidence intervals are a way of expressing how much different they could be. Therefore, they are essential for us to decide whether a result is likely to be true for the whole population or whether it could have occurred by chance. The conventional Forrest plot is very helpful in showing what the confidence intervals mean in terms of interpreting the results (Fig. 3). The error bars show how CIs shrink with increasing population size while the position of the effect estimate square shows the result in terms of effect size.

Two questions you can ask yourself about the confidence intervals:

Do they cross the "line of no difference"? If they do, then the results are not statistically significant. Maybe their sample was too small.
Would your clinical decision be the same if the true value was at the top of the CI range as if it were at the bottom? Is the CI so wide that you cannot rely on the result?

Clinical papers should report confidence intervals around their results. If they do not, be suspicious.

Deciding on relevance

This is the real thorny issue of evidence-based practice for which clinical expertise is paramount. However, you can make the problem more manageable by breaking it down according to the following three-part question:

Are your patients similar to those in the study?
Can your service provide the intervention in the same way as in the trial?
Do the outcomes from the study match up with the ones that matter to you and your patients?

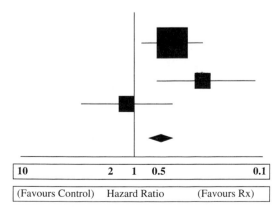

Fig. 3. Confidence intervals.

Patients

The first step is to turn this question around: Is your patient so different from those studied that the results cannot help you? [5] The next step is to think about how much the results can help you. There are a number of ways to frame your thinking:

- What clinical factors would affect your patient's chances of benefiting or suffering a bad outcome?
- Would any of these preclude any benefit from the study intervention?
- Can you estimate your patient's relative chances of benefiting? If you think your patient has, for example, double the risk of those in the study, you might expect them to derive double the absolute benefit.

Interventions

Any benefits the evidence showed for an intervention will only translate to your practice if you can deliver it in a similar way. Therefore, you should consider the following:

- Can you deliver it in your setting?
- Do you need to think about training or service modifications to be able to implement it?
- Will any differences between other aspects of how you manage this type of patient and how they were managed in the study affect the outcomes?
- Does it cost more than the alternative, and are the benefits worth it?

Outcomes

Finally, you need to consider whether the outcomes described in the study are the ones that matter to you and to your patients. You probably decided what they were before you started analyzing the article, but sometimes the process of going through it will change your mind.

Summary

For everyday clinical practice, most surgeons will want to find a reasonable slice of the good evidence on a question very quickly. You should use a simple specific search strategy such as the PubMed clinical query. This is a task that is feasible to fit in between other office jobs. If you are going to publish your results or change your hospital (or national) policy depending on them, you clearly need to be more thorough.

References

[1] Solomon MJ, McLeod RS. Surgery and the randomised controlled trial: past, present and future. Med J Aust 1998;169:380–3.
[2] Taylor I, Sasako M, Lovett B, et al. Randomised trials in surgery: problems and possible solutions. BMJ 2002;324:1448–51.

[3] National Health Service CRD. Accessing the evidence on clinical effectiveness. 2005.

[4] Richardson WS, Wilson MC, Nishikawa J, et al. The well-built clinical question: a key to evidence-based decisions. ACP J Club 1995;123:A12.

[5] Sackett DL, Straus SE, Richardson WS, et al. Evidence-based medicine: how to practise and teach EBM. London: Churchill Livingstone; 2000.

[6] Osheroff JA, Forsythe DE, Buchanan BG, et al. Physicians' information needs: analysis of questions posed during clinical teaching. Ann Intern Med 1991;114:576–81.

[7] Cheng GY. Educational workshop improved information-seeking skills, knowledge, attitudes and the search outcome of hospital clinicians: a randomised controlled trial. Health Info Libr J 2003;20(Suppl 1):22–33.

[8] Bias. *Bandolier* 2000;October:80–2.

[9] Epstein AE, Bigger JT Jr, Wyse DG, et al. Events in the Cardiac Arrhythmia Suppression Trial (CAST): mortality in the entire population enrolled. J Am Coll Cardiol 1991;18:14–9 [erratum: J Am Coll Cardiol 1991;18:888].

[10] Graham DJ, Campen D, Hui R, et al. Risk of acute myocardial infarction and sudden cardiac death in patients treated with cyclo-oxygenase 2 selective and non-selective non-steroidal anti-inflammatory drugs: nested case-control study. Lancet 2005;365:475–81.

[11] Schulz KF, Chalmers I, Hayes RJ, et al. Empirical evidence of bias: dimensions of methodological quality associated with estimates of treatment effects in controlled trials. JAMA 1995;273:408–12.

ELSEVIER
SAUNDERS

Surg Clin N Am 86 (2006) 59–70

SURGICAL
CLINICS OF
NORTH AMERICA

Teaching Evidence-Based Decision-Making

Nick Sevdalis, BSc, MSc, PhD[a],*,
Peter McCulloch, MD, FRCSEd[b]

[a]*Clinical Safety Research Unit, Department of Bio-Surgery & Surgical Technology,
Imperial College, 10th Floor, QEQM, St. Mary's Hospital, South Warf Road,
London, England W2 1NY, UK*
[b]*Nuffield Department of Surgery, John Radcliffe Hospital, University of Oxford,
Headington, Oxford OX3 9DU, England, UK*

Decision-making is a key activity in everyday clinical practice. The selection of diagnostic tests, the development of a management plan, and the choice of how to approach communication with the patient are all decision-making processes. Surgery is a particularly challenging specialty when it comes to decision-making, because of the need to make rapid intraoperative decisions that may have important and irreversible consequences. It is therefore not very surprising that a self-selection process seems to occur when trainees come to choose specialty careers, whereby people who have a personality profile favoring decisiveness are more likely to choose a surgical career [1,2]. Surgeons as a group have "stable extrovert" personality traits, which might be expected to lead them to favor action over contemplation and intuition over calculation (McCulloch et al, submitted for publication, 2004) [3]. Teaching surgeons to make decisions might therefore be seen as an unproductive activity, but persuading them to use evidence properly in so doing may be both challenging and potentially valuable.

Understanding the decision-making process

Decision-making in medicine, as in all other walks of life, is hardly ever accomplished by careful weighing of full and accurate information and objective choice based on clearly defined evaluation of the possible outcomes. It is important to recognize that there is a large number of pressures that may influence a clinical decision. Fig. 1 is an illustrative but not inclusive

---

* Corresponding author.
E-mail address: n.sevdalis@imperial.ac.uk (N. Sevdalis).

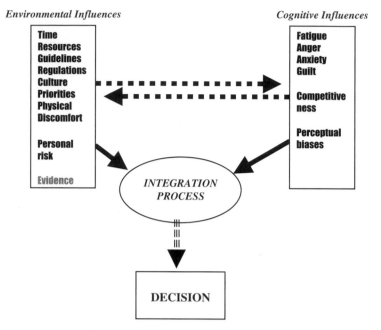

Fig. 1. Influences of clinical decision-making.

list. The relevant evidence should play a central role, but it is unrealistic to expect, or to teach, that it will always be predominant. This is reflected in Sackett's definition of evidence-based medicine as "the integration of best research evidence with clinical expertise and patient values" [4]. Psychological research shows us that in fact there is a great deal more going on even than this (see below).

The characteristics of a decision determine the way people view it. Some of these characteristics are particularly influential in determining whether the decision is easy or difficult, stressful or almost unnoticed. They can be looked on as dimensions of the decision, because their combined influence on the perceived difficulty of the decision is more like a product than a sum. A list of the most important decision dimensions is shown in Box 1, together with a commentary on each. It is interesting to note how each of these affects the decision maker's attitude to considering the available evidence. Time pressure, for example, always make it subjectively more difficult for the clinician to use evidence properly, and irreversibility may have this effect or the opposite one, depending on other factors, including the prior attitude of the clinician.

Influences on decision-making in medicine

There is empirical evidence that humans do not approach decision-making situations in the same manner as a computer system would do.

Box 1. Decision dimensions

- Time pressure: enhances the anxiety of decision-making. Leads to use of error-prone cognitive strategies. Strongly discourages objective evaluation of relevant evidence. These properties are always enhanced by combination with other dimensions.
- Importance: enhances the anxiety of decision-making; can lead to complete inability to decide. If not combined with time pressure, may increase the likelihood of consulting the evidence base. May also increase reliance on experience and intuition.
- Fuzziness: where the decision is not a clear-cut choice between a small number of options, but allows for a range of solutions. May increase or decrease anxiety and subjective difficulty. Effect on the role of evidence may be positive or negative, depending on other factors.
- Reversibility: irreversibility increases decision anxiety and difficulty. Effect on the use of evidence depends on pre-existing attitudes, but many patients and clinicians show an apparently paradoxical reliance on intuition and experience when faced with an irreversible decision.
- Incomplete information: enhances the anxiety of decision-making; can lead to complete inability to decide. Tends to make reliance on objective evidence less likely, because the applicability of the evidence cannot be guaranteed, and judgment is bound to play a greater role.

On the one hand, human decision-making is constrained by the brain's capacity for processing information [5–7], whereas on the other hand, people are not always motivated to seek optimal solutions to problems. This is especially true when decision-makers are tired or distracted, or the stakes are low, so that the decision makers' personal involvement is minimal. The combination of our relatively low information-processing capabilities and low motivation results in the seeking out of "good enough" rather than "optimal" alternatives.

There are at least two classes of influences on individual decision-making processes: external influences and internal influences.

External influences

External influences stem from the human and physical environment where the decisions are actually taken. This class encompasses the following facets.

Physical environment

Levels of temperature, humidity, and ambient noise are important aspects of the work-space that can affect decision-making ability. Where the clinician is exhausted, or made uncomfortable by heat, cold, hunger, pain or illness, decision-making will be more difficult and usually less efficient.

The use of high-tech equipment and computer-based diagnostic tools can often add to the complexity of the decision environment. Empirical research has only recently addressed these features in the medical environment [8].

Human environment

Surgery is a work space where there are a wide range of tasks to be completed, involving interactions among medical subspecialties and support staff. Teamwork in this environment is the rule rather than the exception. The operating theater is an example of the complexities of teamwork that involves at least three subspecialties (nursing, anesthetic, and surgical staff) at various levels of expertise. The role of teamwork and the interaction between different professionals in the delivery of effective health care has recently become a focus of significant research interest [8,9].

Organizational environment

The physical and the human environment are embedded in a broader organizational context, and the relationships between the three are complex. The concepts of organizational culture and climate [10] are constructs that have been developed to account for the obvious but difficult-to-analyze influences of the organization on how individuals and teams within them behave.

To a practicing clinician, the perceived external pressures that influence decision-making are principally time, resources, and the "rules" of the clinical environment. In this latter category there is a hierarchy ranging from the absolute requirements of the legal system and the clinician's ethical code; though protocols and guidelines laid down by hospitals, health organizations and professional bodies; to more nebulous but often equally powerful rules, such as those created by peer expectations and organizational culture ("the way we do it 'round here"). Time is probably the influence that gives us the most common cause for anxiety, but the perceived lack of time in a clinical environment often reflects a situation in which there are several decisions to be made in a given period and insufficient time to consider them all fully. There is therefore a process of prioritization going on constantly in the clinician's mind, often subconsciously. We are aware of the impossibility of doing everything immediately, and a secondary decision-making process of deciding which decisions to make first occurs.

Availability of evidence

The availability or lack of relevant objective evidence is of course also an environmental factor. Its inclusion at the end of this list emphasizes the inevitability of subjective influences on decision-making. What clinicians, together with most other nonpsychologists, often fail to appreciate is that the environmental influences are in many cases less important than inevitable biases introduced by the psychological processes involved in human decision-making.

Internal influences

Internal influences are the second class that affects individual decision-making processes. These stem from the architecture and performance requirements of the human cognitive system. They can be either intrinsic in the system or exogenous to it. Research on the exogenous influences on the cognitive system has shown that people's capacity to process information can be adversely affected by a host of factors, including those below.

Lack of sleep and fatigue

Surgeons in training who hade been deprived of sleep took longer to complete surgical tasks, made more errors, and were more stressed than surgeons who were on call the night before and surgeons who had an undisturbed night's sleep [11]. The Batelle Report [12] provided a conceptual clarification of fatigue and a range of tools for assessing the effects of pilot fatigue on task performance, and its findings were very similar to those of Taffinder and colleagues [11] in terms of the detrimental effects of lack of sleep on people's ability to process information and perform complex tasks.

Time pressure

Time pressure induces stress on the decision-making process independent of the decision itself (which may or may not carry a stress load of its own). Time pressure and stress usually result in cognitive shortcuts and inadequate information processing. They also lead to over-reliance on courses of action that have been effective previously, even when the features of the decision have changed considerably (see Svenson and Maule [13] for a review).

Research on the intrinsic influences on decision-making has demonstrated that, in a wide range of circumstances and decision tasks, people's decision-making processes differ fundamentally from the logical "maximization algorithms" used in computer decision-making software. Some of the findings of this line of research are particularly relevant to medical decision-making (see Chapman and Elstein [14] for a review):

Use of heuristics

From the vast array of possibilities stored in their memory (or in textbooks) people produce judgments on the basis of only a few, readily available categories (the availability heuristic [15]). Any event (eg, a news item) that changes the range of readily available information in memory is likely to affect subsequent decisions based on this information. Diagnoses are an example of medical decisions that are very likely to be affected by availability [16]. A number of other heuristics, such as time discounting (the placing of greater value on rewards which are immediately available), are known to be important in human decision-making, and are well described in the psychology literature [17].

Systematic failure to apply basic rules of probabilistic reasoning correctly to decision problems

People find it hard to reason with information presented to them in a probabilistic format, and this can lead to important errors in clinical thinking. Two examples of this inability are: (1) the neglect of relevant base rate information in favor of irrelevant information [18], and (2) the confusion between a diagnostic tool's sensitivity and specificity when actual data is provided and the patient needs a diagnosis framed in terms of "likelihood" [19]. This can lead to misinterpretation of good objective evidence, and hence to decisions based on false conclusions.

Role of moods and emotions

People produce probabilistic estimates of events in accordance with their current moods. Higher moods are associated with more optimistic estimates and lower moods with more pessimistic ones [20]. An important influence on decision-making is the tendency to try to minimize the regrets that decision-makers will experience as a result of their behavior, especially when they know that the outcomes of non-chosen courses of action will be communicated to them [21]. We think of decisions to act as more our responsibility than decisions not to. This may partly explain why people are apparently more willing to accept the risk of death to their child as a result of a disease than to accept the same outcome as a side effect of a vaccine against the disease, when they themselves would have made the decision to vaccinate (omission bias [22]).

Principles of teaching evidence-based decision-making: content

There are so many effective ways of teaching this subject that any recommendations are bound to be somewhat idiosyncratic and based on personal experience, rather than on objective evidence of superiority. That said, there are some aspects of evidence-based decision-making that will always need to be addressed in any meaningful teaching program, and these have relationships to each other that give an almost inevitable structure to the way in which the whole session develops.

Compiling a list of sources of evidence

This is useful starting point, because it allows people to focus on their own particular environment in a practical way, which will ensure they feel comfortable that what they are doing is straightforward and has value.

Most hospitals in countries that have easy access to computers will be able to connect to a great variety of databases, so in theory they should be able to obtain evidence on any subject easily. In practice, the access that is easily available to the average clinician without specialist computer expertise varies greatly. Clinicians are often unaware of the relevant data sources other than PubMed, and involvement of a librarian or information technology (IT) expert in the session at this point can be very valuable in helping to develop a useful list of resources. One common problem is that abstracts may be freely available on the net, but full-text articles are not, and many libraries cannot offer a retrieval service for full text that is fast enough to be clinically useful. It is, moreover, quite common for hospitals to have extensive links to full-text retrieval services about which the clinicians working there are very poorly informed, and again a librarian can help here. Handouts usually end up in the bin, but a list of potentially useful resources available in the local environment is more likely to be used if it is permanently and prominently displayed somewhere in the working environment (preferably not too far from a computer that can be used to access some of the resources listed). Facing up to the practical difficulties is often a useful basis for launching a discussion on what we can reasonably hope to achieve in our particular workplace. There are ways in which evidence can be use to inform the decision-making process in nearly all hospital environments, but the need for a solution that will work in practice needs to be emphasized. In a typical UK hospital, for example, there is a computer terminal on each ward on which, in theory, access to PubMed is available; however, the terminal is usually in constant use in a busy thoroughfare or nurses station, so planning to search for evidence on it during a ward round is unrealistic.

Influences on decision-making and role of evidence

After setting the scene by defining what resources are actually available in a practical sense, another essential step in teaching evidence-based decision-making is to get the group to appreciate the nature of the obstacles they face. As discussed above, these are both environmental and cognitive, and clinicians are usually much more aware of the former than of the latter. Using brainstorming is an excellent way of getting a realistic list of influences on decisions in the environments the participants experience, but it will very likely need some direction by the moderator.

Because clinicians are not accustomed to examining the mental processes by which they reach their conclusions, and are mostly unfamiliar with the substantial research evidence about cognitive biases, they may well require prompting and the use of examples to consider these seriously. It is very useful to be prepared for this by having some striking examples from psychological research available whose translation into a medical scenario is easy to envisage. Quite often the thought will occur to one of the participants that a search for the evidence on cognitive problems in decision-making would be a good idea. To encourage this while preventing the group from drowning in the extensive literature that exists, facilitators should (1) be able to direct the group to PsycInfo and perhaps one or two other online databases on the psychology literature, and (2) have some recommendations ready on overviews and texts that give a good introduction to the literature while avoiding unnecessary detail.

Appropriate levels of evidence base for decisions in context

The commonest (and most justified) complaint of clinicians about evidence-based medicine in general is the practicality of obtaining and evaluating evidence in time to make a difference to clinical practice. Like the strictures of the Church to avoid sin, unrealistic exhortations to try harder are liable to be counterproductive, generating disillusion and cynicism. A strategy that is more likely to be successful in persuading clinicians to make a sustained change in the way they use evidence is to have a discussion with them about the weight of evidence that is appropriate and practical in different situations. This can be started by suggesting that they write down a usable strategy for using evidence in their clinical decision-making. This should be examined critically, to expose unrealistic expectations and to highlight the features that are important in integrating evidence into practice. It may be helpful to ask group members to imagine themselves on a ward round, in clinic, or in the operating room, and ask them how they could use evidence to make decisions in these contexts. Members will emphasize immediate availability, speed of searching, reliability, conciseness, and ease of interpretation as factors that would make it more likely that they use evidence. Discussion should be directed to ensure the value of using what is already available in "predigested" form, such as existing compilations of systematic reviews (Cochrane, Clinical Evidence) and critically appraised topics (CATS) lists from colleagues and other institutions. It will be useful to challenge assumptions about the prospective use of evidence. Often clinicians who reject the use of evidence in real time because of the practical problems will see the value in noting problems for later analysis in a less pressured environment such as an end-of-round coffee break, a weekly unit meeting or a monthly divisional morbidity and mortality (M & M) meeting. It is important to emphasize that evidence-based decision-making is merely a particular aspect of evidence-based medicine, not a new subject that needs to be mastered alongside the main curriculum.

Discuss tactics on how to acquire evidence at appropriate level

The next stage in discussion evolves almost inevitably from the discussion of defining appropriate levels of evidence for different situations. Provided the group members are reasonably motivated, they should be open to the idea of developing a set of solutions to their own problems in getting and using evidence to inform decision-making. They should be encouraged to record this for later use, so that it can be used as a guide to using evidence support for decisions as a matter of regular policy. Solutions will need to be graded depending on the importance of the decision and the time available. For example, surgeons may feel comfortable with a very simple "quick and dirty" PubMed search for a one-time search after a minor clinical query on the ward round, but would want to do a more formal search and analysis for a decision that was going to change an important aspect of their practice for the foreseeable future, to a full systematic review in cases in which unit policy in an area of particular interest or expertise was at stake. Tactical discussions should be at a very practical level, particularly emphasizing when and how evidence could be referred to in a way that does not disrupt or consume the structure of the working day, and who should be responsible for finding and analyzing it. Groups should be reminded to consider both IT-based solutions such as the use of handheld computers to record and transfer information and link to libraries, the development of a local collection of CATS on which literature searches and critical appraisal have already been carried out, the creation of a custom-made list of evidence links that is widely available to all staff on all computers, and so on; and administrative solutions such as developing a set of evidence-based protocols, or assigning set times to evidence searching at the end of rounds and during or before weekly or monthly unit meetings.

Discuss implementation strategies

Once participants have decided on a system for incorporating evidence into their clinical decision-making, there is a natural tendency to regard the session as complete. It needs to be stressed at this stage that good intentions, in this area as in the rest of life, are not enough. To ensure that the decisions made are integrated into unit practice, it is strongly advisable to develop a unit strategy, write it down, and refer to it at regular, preplanned intervals, most conveniently at Unit meetings. Surgeons will want to design their own strategy, but it should be practical and specific, rather than theoretical and principle-based, so that it is easy for unit members to evaluate their performance against it. An example of how a unit strategy might look is shown in Box 2.

Principles of teaching evidence-based decision-making: teaching methods and tactics

As will be clear from the above, the authors strongly favor interactive group discussion methods for teaching evidence-based medicine in general, and regard them as essential in teaching its application at a practical level. This does require a little time while group dynamics, objectives, and ways of working are developed. It is therefore unwise to try to teach this subject in a 1-hour session. As for all group work, facilitators will need to anticipate

---

Box 2. Implementation policy used by the authors for evidence-based decision-making

1. Arrange to have sources of good, well-packaged evidence installed on the local computer network, and have Internet access in clinics, theaters, and ward rounds.
2. Conduct ward rounds and clinics using evidence in real time when possible.
3. When real-time evidence is not possible, apply evidence retrospectively, either at the end of ward rounds or at a regular monthly audit meeting, using a set protocol.
4. Build up a library of evidence-based decisions in areas of practice in which the same question is likely to come up frequently. These may be recorded as CATS or in other appropriate formats. Place them on the local computer network in an easily accessible format.
5. Place reminders to use evidence, and how to do this, in strategic locations in the workplace.
6. Regularly evaluate use of evidence, and whether it could be improved.

---

the likely problems in group dynamics, and have solutions ready to hand. In surgical teams there is normally a strong element of "power distance" between the permanent staff and the trainees, and standard tactics for dealing with this should be used to ensure that all can contribute usefully and feel comfortable. Pairing off senior and junior members; giving dominant individuals roles in which they have to serve the group, such as minute-keeping; and brainstorming by writing (putting suggestions on slips of paper) are all useful methods. One of the weaknesses of group learning is that its lack of structure means that keeping to a timetable can be difficult, and facilitators will need to divide the session up strictly into phases to ensure that the topics are covered. Role playing in which proposed solutions of evidence finding and analysis are tested in a mock round with a real computer is very useful in "debugging" suggestions and making them more practicable. It is obviously important for the teaching to occur where facilities for online searching are adequate and available exclusively for the use of the group. A librarian who has good knowledge of resource finding on the Web is a very important ally in teaching this subject, and surgeons often value tips (even as handouts) from someone who has content expertise in this area. The extent to which clinicians in a team have control over their own work varies greatly depending on the nature of the health system, but in many if not most sophisticated systems, changes in practice require the sanction of members of a management structure within the hospital. It is therefore very important that the individuals with financial power over decision-making in the surgical unit are made part of the process and invited to the session.

Summary

Evidence-based decision-making is particularly important in surgery, but has special difficulties posed by the nature of the work. To teach it successfully requires an interactive approach with a clinical team whose members are willing to consider it seriously, and to think out practical solutions that fit their work environment. The process of decision-making and the influences on it need to be examined and understood, so that surgeons have a realistic idea of the role evidence can play. The importance of cognitive factors in particular must not be ignored. Strategies developed by the team themselves in the context of this knowledge are more likely to be adopted and found useful. It is important to involve experts in searching for evidence, and members of the management team in the learning process; the former to provide expertise on searching, the latter to ensure that the reasons for proposed changes are understood and treated sympathetically by those who have financial control.

References

[1] DeForge BR, Sobal J. Investigating whether medical students' intolerance of ambiguity is associated with their specialty selections. Acad Med 1991;66(1):49–51.

[2] Gilligan JH, Welsh FK, Watts C, et al. Square pegs in round holes: has psychometric testing a place in choosing a surgical career? A preliminary report of work in progress. Ann R Coll Surg Engl 1999;81(2):73–9.

[3] McGreevy J, Wiebe D. A preliminary measurement of the surgical personality. Am J Surg 2002;184(2):121–5.

[4] Sackett DL, Straus S, Richardson S, et al. Evidence based medicine: how to practice and teach EBM. Edinburgh (UK): Harcourt; 2000.

[5] Simon HA. Rational choice and the structure of the environment. Psychol Rev 1956;63: 129–38.

[6] Simon HA. Models of man. New York: Wiley; 1957.

[7] Simon HA. Models of bounded rationality. Cambridge (MA): The MIT Press; 1997.

[8] Healey AN, Undre S, Vincent CA. Developing observational measures of teamwork in surgery. Supplement on team training and simulation. Qual Saf Health Care 2004;13:i33–40.

[9] Grote G, Zala-Melö E. The effects of different forms of coordination in coping with work load: cockpit versus operating theatre; report on the psychological part of the project. Stuttgart (Germany): Daimler-Benz Corporation; 2004.

[10] Schein EH. Organizational culture and leadership. New York: Wiley; 2004.

[11] Taffinder NJ, McManus IC, Gul Y, et al. Effect of sleep deprivation on surgeons' dexterity on laparoscopy simulator. Lancet 1998;352:1191.

[12] An overview of the scientific literature concerning fatigue, sleep, and the circadian cycle. Batelle Memorial Institute—JIL Information Systems; 1998.

[13] Svenson O, Maule AJ. Time pressure and stress in human judgment and decision-making. New York and London: Plenum Press; 1993.

[14] Chapman GB, Elstein AS. Cognitive processes and biases in medical decision-making. In: Chapman GB, Sonnenberg FA, editors. Decision-making in health care: theory, psychology, and applications. New York: Cambridge University Press; 2000. p. 183–210.

[15] Tversky A, Kahneman D. Judgment under uncertainty: heuristics and biases. Science 1974; 185:1124–31.

[16] Poses RM, Anthony M. Availability, wishful thinking, and physicians' diagnostic judgments for patients with suspected bacteremia. Med Decis Making 1991;11:159–68.

[17] Plous S. The psychology of judgement and decision-making. 1st edition. New York: McGraw Hill; 1993.

[18] Kahneman D, Tversky A. Evidential impact of base rates. In: Kahneman D, Slovic P, Tversky A, editors. Judgment under uncertainty: heuristics and biases. Cambridge (UK): Cambridge University Press; 2004. p. 153–60.

[19] Hoffrage U, Lindsay S, Hertwig R, et al. Communicating statistical information. Science 2000;290:2261–2.

[20] Johnson EJ, Tversky A. Affect, generalization, and the perception of risk. J Pers Soc Psychol 1983;45:20–31.

[21] Zeelenberg M. Anticipated regret, expected feedback and behavioral decision-making. Journal of Behavioral Decision-making 1999;12:93–106.

[22] Ritov I, Baron J. Reluctance to vaccinate: omission bias and ambiguity. Journal of Behavioral Decision-making 1990;3:263–77.

ELSEVIER
SAUNDERS

Surg Clin N Am 86 (2006) 71–90

SURGICAL
CLINICS OF
NORTH AMERICA

Librarians, Surgeons, and Knowledge

Thalia Knight, MA (Rhodes), MA (London), MCLIP[a],*,
Anne Brice, BA (Hons), Dip. Lib., MCLIP[b]

[a]*Library and Information Services, The Royal College of Surgeons of England,
35-43 Lincoln's Inn Fields, London WC2A 3PE, England, UK*
[b]*National Library for Health, Badenoch Building, Old Road Campus,
University of Oxford, Headington, Oxford OX3 7LF, England, UK*

"If knowledge is truly to be 'the enemy of disease,' rather than a bystander, it must be readily available when making clinical decisions, planning research, or writing papers"—W. Summerskill [1]

In the 1990s, as the Internet developed, and with it the growth of electronic publishing, librarians found themselves at the forefront of a new and complex environment that would bring a bewildering array of information directly to clinicians and their patients. The ensuing quantum leap in increased information brought with it new challenges as well, which included the issue of how to identify poor quality or unsafe information published on Web sites. Librarians were quick to realize the need for guidelines in evaluating Web site quality, and were pioneers in setting up evaluated gateways to health information. In the United Kingdom, OMNI (Organising Medical Networked Information) [2] led the way in the 1990s, and has now become part of a larger biomedical science gateway based at the University of Nottingham, called BIOME [3]. (For OMNI internet evaluation guidelines see http://omni.ac.uk/guidelines/eval/.) The exponential increase in the quantity of scientific literature has been well-documented (see, for example, Refs. [4–6]) and is far from being a modern phenomenon [7], although electronic publishing has appeared to make the problem of information management worse. The sheer scale and speed of development of the Internet [8] has precipitated previously unimagined challenges—and opportunities. The simultaneous development of evidence-based health care has provided the library and information science profession generally with an even greater imperative to ensure that the best available knowledge is to hand when needed

* Corresponding author.
   E-mail address: tknight@rcseng.ac.uk (T. Knight).

by clinicians. Yet, for all the advances in technology, this remains a holy grail to be sought by everyone in the information chain.

Why is it so difficult for not just for surgeons, but for health care professionals generally, to find the evidence needed for decision-making?

Information overload

With the increase in electronic mail, bulletin boards, discussion lists, and other new electronic sources such as Really Simple Syndication (RSS), information overload is a reality for all health professionals on a day-to-day basis. As previously mentioned, there is the mind-boggling amount of information available on the Internet, which the increasing sophistication of search engines such as Google and Yahoo has exacerbated; users frequently also lack the skills needed to manage the information deluge effectively [9].

Problems with the scientific literature

Furthermore there are also problems of quality because of poor research design; faulty indexing [10,11], and even fraud [12,13], as well as publication delay and bias of various kinds [14–17].

Personal and organizational challenges

Health practitioners have challenges to face, on individual and organizational levels, affecting their ability to retrieve and store relevant, timely, good-quality information. We know from research that the way that individuals approach the search for information, their information behavior, can affect what they find, and therefore what they use [18].

Poorly designed information systems

Given that many information systems, including institutional intranets, are poorly organized, with little consistency or common standards of presentation and quality of content, it is not a surprise that finding the evidence remains a complex and difficult problem, in an increasingly time-poor working environment. Requiring busy health professionals to relearn how to use existing systems whenever the interface or the system itself is upgraded, or to take on new systems that need an investment of time to learn, adds to their burden.

Authentication and e-license barriers

Access via password/identification to licensed resources or some other form of authentication such as the Athens [19] system, widely in use in the United Kingdom within the National Health Service (NHS) as well as higher education and professional bodies, may act as a practical and psychological barrier when users are faced with needing to remember a plethora of passwords or personal identification (PIN) numbers. Authentication by internet provider (IP) address range only partly addresses the issue when health professionals need to access content outside the licensed site (eg, at home, at a conference).

Lack of access to computer equipment

Even in the developed world, adequate access to computer equipment and to sufficient bandwidth, especially within the hospital setting, can be difficult. Networks and hardware are subject to technical and operating failure and require ongoing maintenance, which may be subject to budgetary constraints. Internal security (firewalls and the like) can all also inadvertently cause problems at the point of access. All too often proprietary systems are installed that are not interoperable, creating further barriers to collaboration and knowledge sharing.

General barriers reviewed

The major general barriers to accessing the evidence could be listed as follows:

Lack of time and skills
Information overload
Variable quality in indexing and applying metadata
New, important information sources arriving all the time
New systems lack standardization and require time to learn.
Getting hold of information from multiple sources and in multiple formats requires good supporting infrastructure that may not be there yet.
Systems that are in place are likely to be proprietary and probably lack interoperability, creating further barriers.

What is the role of the information specialist in twenty-first century health care?

How can the skills of librarians help overcome the information problems encountered by the health practitioner and contribute to evidence-based practice in particular, and thus to improvements in health and well being generally? What could be the role of an information specialist within the surgical team?

First we need to take account of current developments within the information profession itself in relation to the health profession and evidence-based practice, and emerging understanding of what constitutes surgical knowledge in practice.

The "informationist" debate

By 2000, clinicians themselves had begun to recognize the paradigm shifts in research, audit, and teaching brought about by the advent of electronic publishing in general, as well as in relation to biomedical information and clinical practice within developing clinical informatics systems.

During the 1990s, there were two parallel developments that impacted on the practice of evidence-based medicine (EBM). The first has been the rise of biomedical informatics as biomedical research has seen the spectacular growth of huge scientific datasets, along with the pervasive use of information and communication technologies (ICT) in scientific research, including creating and storing medical images and data in ways previously only imagined. The second has been the use of ICT in health care administration, most notably in North America, but now growing fast in Europe and the Pacific rim nations. This includes the development of electronic patient and health care records, alongside hospital and primary care systems for recording the results of investigations, the prescribing of drugs, clinic bookings, and so on. The need to integrate knowledge with health care systems is evidenced by the ability of physicians in many US hospitals, for example, to call up the results of laboratory tests and online pharmacopoeias, as well as summaries of evidence, via their clinic or ward computers or on their handheld computers. In the United Kingdom, knowledge support system projects aim to integrate medical knowledge within the developing National Care Record system [20]. The Web site http://www.connectingforhealth.nhs.uk/ contains up-to-date information on this and related developments within the NHS.

In a frequently cited article published in the *Annals of Internal Medicine* in June 2000, Davidoff and Florance called for the development of a new professional, whom they called an "informationist" [21]. Much debate followed (see for example, refs. [22–24]), particularly in relation to existing "clinical librarian" models; what new training, knowledge, skills and attributes were needed; financial models required to support an "informationist" service; implementation and promotional activities; and how to evaluate the impact of a "clinical informationist" service. The idea of a "clinical (medical) librarian" is not new [25–28] and, indeed, the model is currently under debate and development [29–34] on both sides of the Atlantic.

Summerskill [1] points out that with the development of systematic reviews and critical appraisal as part of the practice of evidence-based health care has come "… the realisation that not all clinicians will need or want to do literature searches and critical appraisal. … To avoid the danger of superficial results, researchers, practitioners, and managers need ready access to experts who can undertake reliable searches, and are conversant with the many databases that different clients require." Summerskill also notes that although clinical teams now include many professions allied to health, it is still rare to find a librarian or "informationist." A survey of UK clinical librarians performed in June 2005 identified only 25 clinical librarians work-ing across the United Kingdom "offering clinical librarian or similar out-reach information services to staff in hospital settings" [33]. In their paper on the "Evolution of a Mature Clinical Informationist Model," Guise and colleagues [34] discuss the history of the clinical medical librarianship model, and also note that in the United States too, it "met with limited up-take." Medical librarians have from the beginning been quick to recognize that they have a unique role in supporting evidence-based health care, both in exploiting technology to better organize, manage, and deliver the knowledge base, and in helping to skill practitioners in order for them to ac-cess and use evidence.

Eskind Biomedical Library case study

The work done at the Eskind Biomedical Library (EBL) at Vanderbilt University Medical Centre (VUMC) by Guise and her staff in developing Davidoff and Florance's idea of a clinical informationist is predicated on "integrating expert information provision with informatics systems" [34]. Thus, the highly trained clinical informationists at EBL are not solely ac-tive members of health care teams carrying out literature searches, provid-ing summaries of evidence, and providing advanced information filtering to the staff they support. They have also begun proactively to integrate the evidence-related services into the internal electronic health care record system in response to patient-care questions sent directly to them via "information baskets." Because they are seen to be an integral part of the care delivery teams, they also have to "sign and agree to abide by the same stringent confidentiality measures as clinicians for accessing pa-tient information" [34]. In order further to support the management of common conditions, the EBL clinical informationists have also provided links to nationally recognized guidelines that are dynamically generated by mapping them to the International Classification of Diseases, 9th Revision, Clinical Modification Codes (ICD-9-CM) [35]. They have also created a Pathway Literature Locator database where their "expert, topic-specific search strategies as well as librarians' overall analyses for path-ways topics" are stored, ready to provide automatically updated access to evidence when next required. Guise agrees with Summerskill and others [25,28] that the effectiveness of this type of approach still needs to be for-mally demonstrated. The EBL has therefore been funded by the National Library of Medicine in Bethesda, Maryland to carry out a 3-year evalu-ation of their Clinical Informatics Consult Service's impact on clinical practice and decision-making at VUMC. They predict that the "advanced skills and forward-thinking mentality of informationists make logical the next step of integrating them into clinical software development (infor-matics) teams" [34].

A systemic approach to knowledge management

The experience of the EBL fits with the conclusions drawn by Bali and co-workers [36] in relation to their research into the key issues surrounding the incorporation of the knowledge management paradigm in health care. From a UK perspective they examined the impact of ideas such as clinical governance, EBM, model of integrated patient pathways, and community health information networks in comparison with the alternative ideas offered by knowledge management. They concluded that, "Modern IT [information technology] applications in health care are not sufficient in meeting the information needs of current health care institutions as they lack the ability to deliver precise, accurate and contextual information to the desired caregiver at the desired time." They also believe that "any potential solution has to come from a domain that synergistically combines people, organizational processes and technology" [36]. A systematic review performed in 2004 by Coomarasamy and Khan [37] aimed to "evaluate the effects of standalone versus clinically integrated teaching in evidence-based medicine on various outcomes in postgraduates." They concluded that real change only occurs when EBM teaching is integrated into clinical practice, and acknowledge that this will "require a sustained effort well beyond standalone instruction." This finding adds to the case that continues to be built for a systemic approach to the task of providing access to the best available knowledge.

In 2000, the OpenClinical group based at CancerUK's laboratories in London published a white paper on *The medical knowledge crisis and its solution through knowledge management* [38]. This white paper resulted in the establishment of an internationally supported Web portal for information about developments in the field of medical knowledge management: http://www.openclinical.org. In summary it concluded categorically, among other things, that

It is now humanly impossible for unaided health care professionals to possess all the knowledge needed to deliver medical care with the efficacy and safety made possible by current scientific knowledge.
This can only get worse in the postgenomic era.
A potential solution to the knowledge crisis is the adoption of rigorous methods and technologies for knowledge management.
Awareness and understanding of these methods is not widespread, and many of the technologies that currently exist are not designed to be compatible with others or interoperable.

By 2000, there was clearly consensus that only a collaborative systemic approach stands any chance of solving these challenges to medical knowledge management.

Such a systemic approach has been taken by the National Knowledge Service [39] that was set up within the NHS in the United Kingdom, following the government's response to the outcome of the inquiry into cardiothoracic surgery at Bristol Royal Infirmary. Paragraph 13 of the Secretary of State's response promised "from April 2003, a National Knowledge Service (NKS) for the NHS to support the delivery of high quality information for patients and staff" [40]. The whole system approach being taken is summarized in Fig. 1, a diagram from the National Knowledge Service Web site: http://www.nks.nhs.uk/. See also the complementary pilot Web site http://www.nelh.nhs.uk/kmresearch.

Some idea of the impact of this work program is described by Plaice and Kitch [41]. They note that "Successfully applied, knowledge management is the creation of an environment, an infrastructure and processes that enable the achievement of these (among other) objectives. This indeed makes it clear why some prefer the phrase 'knowledge mobilisation' rather than 'knowledge management'". Indeed "knowledge mobilisation" is the preferred way of understanding the process that the NKS has begun to set in place through its workstreams. This includes the development of the National Library for Health (http://www.nlh.nhs.uk), with its specialist libraries created around communities of practice.

Reflecting on their experience of embedding knowledge within the NHS in the Southwest of England, Plaice and Kitch [41] feel that their experience has taught them "that information professionals have the capacity to understand and demonstrate the importance of a 'whole systems approach' and some of the ways in which knowledge can be harnessed to move the organization forward." A "Specialist Library for Knowledge Management,"

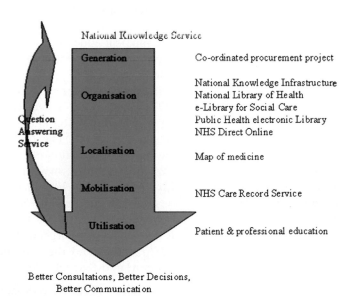

Fig. 1. Activities of the UK National Knowledge Service, © 2004 National Knowledge Service. (*From* http://www.nks.nhs.uk; with permission.)

which "aims to support a knowledge-sharing culture within the National Health Service," is also available via the National Library for Health: http://libraries.nelh.nhs.uk/knowledgemanagement/. A "Specialist Library for Surgery, Theaters and Anesthesia" is under construction and will become publicly available in 2006. Information on the project is available via the Web site of The Royal College of Surgeons of England [42]. As a precursor to this project, an information needs analysis was performed by Nicholas and colleagues [43] to discover what knowledge and information was needed by operating theater staff in an NHS Hospital Trust. Their findings confirmed some of the general factors enumerated above on the difficulties of finding evidence (eg, issues of access; the factors under personal and organizational challenges as well as digital literacy). Nicholas and coworkers [43] discovered that the theater staff, including surgeons, supported the idea of a specialist library that would meet their needs, and that it had the potential to be not merely a digital resource but a digital catalyst.

What kinds of knowledge do surgeons need?

Information professionals need to have some understanding of the particular knowledge needs of surgeons at all stages in their surgical career path in order to be better placed to develop the services that meet those needs. In certain respects surgeons are simply "doctors with knives," and their clinical information needs are no different from the information needs of clinicians generally; however, as other articles in this issue have demonstrated, surgery also faces unique problems in relation to developing a clinical evidence base of knowledge.

In the United Kingdom, postgraduate medical education is undergoing profound changes in its organization, delivery, and assessment as a result of the Government's "Modernising Medical Careers" program (http://www.mmc.nhs.uk). New curricula are being developed for specialty training that will be implemented in August, 2007. This process is overseen by the newly established independent statutory body, the Postgraduate Medical Education Training Board (http://www.pmetb.org.uk). The four surgical colleges of the British Isles are collaborating on the creation of the first national surgical curriculum that is also Web-based (http://www.iscp.ac.uk). Information on the development of this approach has been described by De Cossart and Fish [44,45]. Drawing on research into professional practice and its relationship to tacit as well as explicit knowledge, De Cossart and Fish have explicated a map of practice knowledge for surgeons [46]. They believe that curriculum developers need to understand the wide range of kinds of knowledge that surgeons draw upon, and that includes

Propositional knowledge—this is factual (medical/surgical) knowledge.

Procedural knowledge—this is knowing how to do things.

Intuition—this gives the appearance of informed action without the attendant thought, but it often nudges professionals to investigate something further.

Sensory/embodied knowledge—this involves developing "a good (safe) pair of hands" or "a good eye."

Tacit knowledge—this is propositional or procedural knowledge that has become so embedded in practice that it is invisible.

Professional judgment—this is at the heart of a professional practitioner's practice. [45]

The Intercollegiate Surgical Curriculum developers have also drawn on the pioneering work done by The Royal College of Physicians and Surgeons of Canada in its CanMEDS Project [47,48], and now adopted internationally as a basis for describing the generic skills clinicians have to develop. The CanMEDS 2005 Physician Competency Framework document [49] describes the core competencies based on a series of interrelated roles required to develop the central role of "medical expert" for all medical, including surgical, specialists. The medical expert's roles encompass those of

Communicator
Collaborator
Manager
Health advocate
Scholar
Professional

This framework includes the role of "scholar" in recognition of the fact that professional medical practice requires "a lifelong commitment to reflective learning, as well as the creation, dissemination, application and translation of medical knowledge" [49]. The CanMEDS Project identifies interlinked "key" and "enabling" competencies associated with each role. A key competency for physicians as "medical experts" is to be able to "Establish and maintain clinical knowledge, skills and attitudes appropriate to their practice" [49]. The linked enabling competencies include the abilities to

- Apply knowledge of the clinical, socio-behavioral, and fundamental biomedical sciences relevant to the physician's specialty
- Apply lifelong learning skills of the scholar role to implement a personal program to keep up-to-date, and enhance areas of professional competence

The role of scholar has the key competencies of being able to

- Critically evaluate information and its sources, and apply this appropriately to practice decisions

- Contribute to the creation, dissemination, application and translation of new medical knowledge and practices

The linked enabling competences to achieve this are described, among others, as being able to

- Describe the principles of critical appraisal
- Critically appraise retrieved evidence to address a clinical question
- Integrate critical appraisal conclusions into clinical care
- Describe the principles of research and scholarly inquiry
- Pose a scholarly question
- Conduct a systematic search for evidence
- Select and apply appropriate methods to address the question

What kinds of support do health information professionals provide?

Health information professionals stand to have a more explicitly recognized role in the future by assisting clinicians and by implication, surgeons, in acquiring the generic competencies noted above that involve the knowledge, skills, and experience already part of the information professional's tool kit. Traditionally they have provided resources to support the "propositional" and "procedural" aspects of surgical knowledge, and they increasingly find themselves assisting in helping to document and make accessible "tacit knowledge" as it is made explicit by surgical educators and surgeons in practice; whether via curriculum development, through increasingly sophisticated methods of assessment of competence in surgical practice, or through the multiprofessional dialogue of the surgical team.

By supporting informed and timely decision-making, knowledge services also save time for health professionals, minimize information overload, and reduce risk and unnecessary expenditure, thereby delivering cost-benefits. Effective knowledge services should be available to support informed health care decision-making by health workers, patients, and the public, as well as to facilitate work-based learning and continuing professional development.

In sum, health information professionals are able to help surgeons in the following areas:

Keeping professionally updated
Supporting practice, policies, and procedures
Support at individual, team, and organizational levels
Support for knowledge management services
Support for work-based and lifelong learning, training, and research

Keeping professionally updated

Most clinicians will have experience of journals clubs, which are frequently supported directly and indirectly by their local health library. Other activities performed in support of this aim by librarians include

- Alerting staff to news and information from journals, research, and briefings
- Alerting staff to news and policy developments from within the organization
- Delivering subject-based alerting and awareness services
- Training in and encouraging making optimum use of electronic current awareness services provided by the National Library for Health in the United Kingdom, via PubMed, by the National Library of Medicine (NLM), by local academic medical libraries, or by professional medical bodies

Supporting practice, policies and procedures

With the growing acceptance of EBM, librarians and information scientists are increasingly involved in helping to deliver high quality health care and clinical effectiveness by

- Raising awareness of sources of evidence
- Facilitating access to evidence
- Disseminating information about best practice (guidelines, protocols)
- Expert literature searching
- Undertaking critical appraisal
- Preparing synopses
- Disseminating knowledge about applying evidence in practice

Support at an individual, team, and organizational level

By creating an organizational information node that is responsive to user needs and requirements, librarians can

- Alert users to new knowledge
- Collect and synthesize information from multiple sources
- Index and organize information so that it is easy to find
- Help users navigate the knowledge base
- Search and filter information from multiple sources
- Teach effective use of information resources and personal bibliographic software
- Negotiate access to licensed resources
- Obtain and deliver information direct to the user

Support for knowledge management services

Knowledge supports organizational planning, policy development, project work, and patient care. Many clinical and nonclinical professionals working in allied fields, including health librarians and information specialists, are coming together, whether through research projects or government funded initiatives, to

- Support organizational development through advice and project work

- Contribute to knowledge management programs
- Advise on knowledge management techniques; explore techniques such as knowledge harvesting
- Develop/contribute to intranets and external Web sites
- Develop local electronic information resources
- Contribute local information to national electronic resources
- Support the integration of evidence into the electronic record throughout the patient journey.

Much of this work involves connecting people to people:

- Making corporate (hospital, clinic, health service etc) knowledge and records accessible
- Giving access to knowledge derived from research as well as from experience
- Systematic dissemination of national and local policy and guidance
- Facilitating e-groups, networks, communities of practice, and learning sets
- Providing tailored services and knowledge signposting

Support for work-based and lifelong learning, training, and research

Heath information professionals are already focused on delivering services to support work-based and lifelong learning, training, and research by providing the content of the knowledge base as follows:

- Ready access to up-to-date printed, audiovisual, and electronic resources
- Enabling access to e-learning resources
- Providing reference, stock lending, reservation and renewal services
- Signposting users to specialized resources
- Facilitating document delivery services and developing digital document delivery
- Using quality criteria to select information and learning resources on internet gateways and information portals such as BIOME and similar resources

They use this knowledge base to provide information services:

- Enquiry services, including mediated searching services
- Tailoring services to meet the needs and preferences of different user groups
- Widening participation; provision of information to all clinical and non-clinical health and social care staff
- Delivering information services at the point of care in clinics, on wards, and in operating theaters
- Delivering information services in the workplace to health care administrators

- Enhancing the value of nationally produced resources by adding local knowledge on intranets
- Directing users to national and local services

The health library as a "knowledge nexus"

As the medical profession generally has had to respond to the impact of new technologies affecting health care and changes in the delivery of medical education, medical libraries have also had to respond to these changes. Lindberg and Humphreys [50] postulate some of changes that are likely to be in place by 2015, noting especially the impact of the digital revolution on end-user expectations and behavior. A study had been performed in 2000 by Rindfleisch [51] on the impact of digital materials on the future roles of health science libraries, which anticipated much of what Lindbergh and Humphreys predict.

The trends emerging by 2000 have been confirmed by a recent study performed by Kronenfeld [52], who sees health libraries becoming a "knowledge nexus" thanks to the digital revolution. He documents reports published in the United States that have investigated issues of quality in health care, noting that one of the "major barriers to the practice of a higher quality of care is inadequate systems and resources to support the effective use of evidence in health care" [52]. This is a matter of increasing concern, given "the emergence of an information infrastructure that cuts the tie between the library and the physical location of knowledge-based information (KBI)." Clinicians are increasingly expected to be able to access KBI at the point of care to support evidence-based practice, regardless of the type of clinical setting. Kronenfeld notes that this access "may have an increasing legal significance, if it becomes a recognized component of the standard of care from a malpractice standpoint" [52]. A significant corollary to this development noted by Kronenfeld and others [53–55] is the need for research on how most effectively to achieve a "high level of clinicians' competencies in information literacy by the time of their graduation" [52].

Information literacy and access to knowledge

Information literacy is not the same as "IT skills"; rather, it includes a set of higher order knowledge skills that require IT skills as a basis. The skills needed to underpin the "lifelong commitment to reflective learning" identified by the CanMEDS project as a requirement of good medical practice depend on a person being not merely skilled in the use of IT equipment and standard applications, but also, far more importantly, in being "information literate." McGill University in Montreal, Canada runs a course called "Mastering medical information: an introduction to information literacy in the health sciences" Details can be found at http://www.health.library. mcgill.ca/course/infolit.htm.

What is information literacy? Lorie Kloda [56] defines it succinctly: "Information literacy is the set of skills needed to find, retrieve, analyze and use information."

This definition neatly encapsulates the enabling competencies for the scholar as user of the evidence and knowledge base already described, and is relevant to the propositional, procedural, and professional knowledge identified by De Cossart and Fish [45].

From the mid-1990s especially, library services had frequently found themselves as providers of IT skills training, both through the development of formal courses, but also informally as a safe environment within which users unfamiliar with technology could find safe and consistent support and help. What had become apparent was that library users lacked the necessary understanding and skills in using new technology, and therefore lacked the ability to access the new digital information world. Often this included the not-to-be-underestimated psychological barrier of a lack of keyboarding skills, frequently perceived, particularly by senior doctors, to be a purely secretarial skill. There were of course, also other barriers to other clinicians through the lack of access to computer equipment in the workplace.

As the general level of IT skills rose within the health care community, and initiatives such as the European Computer Driving License came into being, libraries are now increasingly leaving IT skills training per se to others, and concentrating instead on what they would see as their true mission. This includes providing information literacy training in the context of their support for traditional learning, e-learning, and research; developing the digital resources to support multiple clinical and research activities; expert searching; helping to teach critical appraisal; and developing knowledge management strategies and activities within their organizations.

Library and information professional bodies in the United States (the Association of College and Research Libraries [ACRL]), Australia (Council of Australian University Librarians [CAUL]), and in the United Kingdom (Society of College, National and University Libraries [SCONUL]) have all produced standards or models for information literacy [57]. SCONUL produced the "Seven Pillars of Information Literacy," which its Advisory Committee on Information Literacy is developing [58]. Seven headline skills were identified, along with two fundamental building blocks of basic library skills plus IT skills at the base. Between the base and the apex of information literacy (the goal being the competent information literate person) are the seven headline skills and attributes, "… the iterative practice of which leads from being a competent user to the expert level of reflection and critical awareness of information as an intellectual resource" [58].

The exponential increase in the volume of biomedical literature in the second half of the twentieth century, coupled with the digital revolution in scientific publishing referred to above, meant that bibliographic instruction has been part of the activity of health librarians, particularly in the academic sector, for decades. The rise of "problem-based learning" (PBL) within medical schools was seen early on as an opportunity for librarians to work with medical faculty to integrate information-seeking skills and activities into a problem-based curriculum [59–61]. "Finding the evidence" skills training to support evidence-based practice is, therefore, also simply part of the wider information literacy skills issue that is rising up the agenda for information professionals who support training and education in all walks of life.

There has also long been recognition of the need for librarians to be trained to teach, or at least to be given, the skills required for effective user instruction. In a recent review of changes facing the information profession, Palmer [62] notes that, of all emerging trends,

> ... teaching was regarded as the most expanded activity and the one that had changed the most. Linked to the education of users is the need to keep abreast of—and respond to changes in—educational practice. Thus in health there has been a trend towards problem-based learning and this has required librarians to acquaint themselves with the basics of educational theory and to learn new ways of imparting knowledge and information.

Health librarians and information specialists worldwide have risen successfully to the challenge of providing Web-based resources and training courses, frequently in collaboration with their health care colleagues (for examples, see Refs. [63–72]). These are aimed at training anyone interested in EBM in:

- The population/intervention/comparison/outcome(s) (PICO) and population/exposure/outcome(s) (PEO) method for asking an answerable question
- Learning how to conduct an appropriate literature search, including an understanding of Boolean logic and operators
- Gaining understanding of MeSH (Medical Subject Headings—a thesaurus developed by the National Library of Medicine in the United States that is used to index articles in the MEDLINE database, best known as PubMed but available in other forms)
- Learning about the Cochrane Library and other databases important to the practice of EBM
- Learning more generally about published and unpublished resources, and how to go about searching for these
- Learning how to carry out critical appraisal of the literature as part of the systematic review process
- Learning how to use personal bibliographic software (eg, Endnote; Reference Manager, and the like)

Forms of training available generally include

- Structured group tutorials, which are the most widely used form of training—many of which will be a course that in turn is part of a curriculum

- One-on-one training in the use of specific databases or using the Internet more effectively—these sessions may need to have a prearranged appointment.
- Online Web-based training—the provision of online materials is increasingly used to supplement group and individual instruction.

Some of these "new ways of imparting knowledge" have included the development by librarians of Web sites devoted to signposting resources for EBM and creation of interactive Web sites for self-directed learning, including, for example, the development of a PICOmaker for learning how to construct a question that can be turned into a search strategy [73]. The PICOmaker application is part of a larger section by the University of Alberta Libraries' "PDA Zone," aimed at delivering content to users of handheld devices.

Future roles for health libraries

This article has outlined the increasingly diverse roles undertaken by information professionals in support of the surgical team's knowledge needs for evidence-based practice. Such information professionals may be called "clinical informationists," "information scientists," "information specialists," or "librarians." The role titles are indicative of the ferment of change brought about by the digital revolution, and of the continuing determination of health information professionals to rise to the challenges involved in supporting surgeons and everyone in the surgical team, as they endeavor to provide the best possible care for their patients.

Libraries as we know them have changed, and are changing [74–77]. The scholarly communications process is also undergoing profound transformation. Libraries of the future are being reshaped in response to changes in [77]

- The economics of information
- Advances in computing and communications
- Global information policies
- Changes in the nature of teaching, research, and scholarship

In the future we can expect health libraries in particular to be

- Centers of evidence
- Libraries without walls
- Centers of instruction in which to learn skills as well as access knowledge
- Filters
- Centers for research and development

References

[1] Summerskill W. Literature searches: look before you leap. The Lancet 2005;366:13–4.
[2] OMNI. http://omni.ac.uk/about/. Accessed October 19, 2005.

[3] BIOME. http://biome.ac.uk/about/. Accessed October 19, 2005.

[4] Wyatt J. Use and sources of medical knowledge. The Lancet 1991;338:1368–73.

[5] Wyatt J. Clinical knowledge and practice in the information age: a handbook for health professionals. London: Royal Society of Medicine; 2001.

[6] Zipser J. MEDLINE to PubMed and beyond. Presented at the Health Sciences Library Association of New Jersey and New York-New Jersey Chapter of MLA Joint Meeting. Princeton, New Jersey, December 8, 1998. Available at: http://www.nlm.nih.gov/bsd/historypresentation.html. Accessed October 18, 2005.

[7] Price DJ de Solla. Little science, big science. New York: Columbia University Press; 1963.

[8] Caslon Analytics net metrics and statistics guide (version of February 2005). Available at: http://www.caslon.com.au/metricsguide2.htm. Accessed October 18, 2005.

[9] Wilson TD. Information overload: implications for healthcare services. Health Informatics Journal 2001;7(2):112–7.

[10] McDonald S, Lefebvre C, Clarke M. Identifying reports of controlled trials in the BMJ and The Lancet. BMJ 1996;313:1116–7.

[11] Hopewell S, Clarke M, Lusher A, et al. A comparison of handsearching versus MEDLINE searching to identify reports of randomized controlled trials. Stat Med 2002;21(11):1625–34.

[12] Lock S. Fraud in medicine. BMJ 1988;296:376–7.

[13] White C. Suspected research fraud: difficulties of getting at the truth. BMJ 2005;331:281–8.

[14] Dubben HH, Beck-Bornholdt HP. Systematic review of publication bias in studies on publication bias. BMJ 2005;331:433–4.

[15] Stern JM, Simes RJ. Publication bias: evidence of delayed publication in a cohort study of clinical research projects. BMJ 1997;315:640–5.

[16] Hirsch L. Randomized clinical trials: what gets published, and when? Can Med Assoc J 2004; 170(4):481–3.

[17] Moher D, Fortin P, Jadad AR, et al. Completeness of reporting of trials published in languages other than English: implications for conduct and reporting of systematic reviews. The Lancet 1996;347:363–6.

[18] Wilson TD. Information-seeking behaviour and the digital information world. European Science Editing 2004;30(3):77–80.

[19] Available through http://www.athens.ac.uk. Accessed October 18, 2005.

[20] Available at: http://www.connectingforhealth.nhs.uk/delivery/programmes/nhscrs. Accessed October 18, 2005.

[21] Davidoff F, Florance V. The informationist: a new health profession? Ann Intern Med 2000; 132(12):996–8.

[22] Various authors. [Letters in response to article cited in Ref. 21]. Ann Intern Med 2001;134(3): 251–2.

[23] Plutchak TS. Informationists and librarians. Bull Med Libr Assoc 2000;88(4):391–2.

[24] Shipman JP, Cunningham DJ, Holst R, et al. The informationist conference: report. J Med Libr Assoc 2002;90(4):458–64.

[25] Cimpl K. Clinical medical librarianship: a review of the literature. Bull Med Libr Assoc 1985; 73(1):21–8.

[26] Urquhart CJ, Hepworth JB. Comparing and using assessments of the value of information to clinical decision-making. Bull Med Libr Assoc 1996;84(4):482–9.

[27] Giuse NB. Advancing the practice of clinical medical librarianship. Bull Med Libr Assoc 1997;85(4):437–8.

[28] Giuse NB. Clinical medical librarianship: the Vanderbilt experience. Bull Med Libr Assoc 1998;86(3):412–6.

[29] Wagner KC, Byrd GD. Evaluating the effectiveness of clinical medical librarian programs: a systematic review of the literature. J Med Libr Assoc 2004;94(1):14–33.

[30] Sargeant SJE, Harrison J. Clinical librarianship in the UK: temporary trend or permanent profession? Part I: a review of the role of the clinical librarian. Health Info Libr J 2004; 21(3):173–81.

[31] Harrison J, Sargeant SJE. Clinical librarianship in the UK: temporary trend or permanent profession? Part II: present challenges and future opportunities. Health Info Libr J 2004; 21(4):220–6.

[32] Ward L. A survey of UK clinical librarianship: February 2004. Health Info Libr J 2004;22(1): 26–34.

[33] Ward L. Survey of UK clinical librarians June 2005. Final report and contribution to the audit of rapid response clinical question answering services in England and Wales 2005. Available at: http://www.le.ac.uk/li/lgh/library/UKClinicalLibrariansJune2005.doc. Accessed October 19, 2005.

[34] Guise NB, Koonge TY, Jerome RN, et al. Evolution of a mature clinical informationist model. J Am Med Inform Assoc 2005;12(3):249–55.

[35] International Classification of Diseases, 9th revision, Clinical Modification Codes (ICD-9-CM). Available at: http://www.cdc.gov/nchs/about/otheract/icd9/abticd9.htm. Accessed October 18, 2005.

[36] Bali RK, Dwivedi A, Naguib R. Issues in clinical knowledge management: revisiting health-care management. Idea Group Inc., 2005. Available at: http://www.idea-group.com/downloads/excerpts/Bali01.pdf. Accessed October 21, 2005.

[37] Coomarasamy A, Khan KS. What is the evidence that postgraduate teaching in evidence-based medicine changes anything? A systematic review. BMJ 2004;329:1017–21.

[38] Open clinical white paper. The medical knowledge crisis and its solution through knowledge management. Available at: http://www.openclinical.org/docs/whitepaper.pdf. Accessed October 25, 2005.

[39] National Knowledge Service Web site. Available at: http://www.nks.nhs.uk. Accessed October 25, 2005.

[40] Learning from Bristol. The Department of Health's response to the Report of the Public Inquiry Into Children's Heart Surgery at the Bristol Royal Infirmary 1984–1995. Cm 5363. London: Department of Health; 2002. Available from the Publications Library on the Department of Health Web site: http://www.dh.gov.uk/PublicationsAndStatistics/Publications/fs/en. Accessed October 18, 2005.

[41] Plaice C, Kitch P. Embedding knowledge management in the NHS south-west: pragmatic first steps for a practical concept. Health Info Libr J 2003;20:75–85.

[42] Specialist Library for Surgery, Theatres and Anaesthesia. Available at: http://www.rcseng.ac.uk/library/projects/specialistlibrary.html. Accessed October 18, 2005.

[43] Nicholas D, Williams P, Smith A, et al. The information needs of perioperative staff: a preparatory study for a proposed specialist library for theatres (NeLH). Health Info Libr J 2005; 22(1):35–43.

[44] De Cossart L, Fish D. A first curriculum framework for surgical SHOs designed by The Royal College of Surgeons of England. Ann R Coll Surg Engl 2004;86:309–11.

[45] Fish D. The educational thinking behind The Royal College of Surgeons of England's first curriculum framework. Ann R Coll Surg Engl 2004;86:312–5.

[46] De Cossart L, Fish D. Cultivating a thinking surgeon: new perspectives on clinical teaching, learning and assessment. Shrewsbury (UK): tfm Publishing Ltd.; 2005.

[47] Frank JR, Jabbour M, Tugwell P, et al. Skills for the new millenium: report of the societal needs working group, CanMEDS 2000 Project. Ann R Coll Physicians Surg Can 1996;29: 206–16.

[48] CanMEDS 2000. Extract from the CanMEDS 2000 Project Societal Needs Working Group Report. Med Teach 2000;22(6):549–54.

[49] The Royal College of Physicians and Surgeons of Canada. The CanMEDS 2005 Physician Competency Framework. Available at: http://rcpsc.medical.org/canmeds/CanMEDS2005/index.php. Accessed October 24, 2005.

[50] Lindberg DAB, Humphreys BL. 2015—the future of medical libraries. N Engl J Med 2005; 352:1067–70.

[51] Rindfleisch TCW. W(h)ither health science libraries: preliminary study of the dynamics and effects of digital materials use on the future roles of health science libraries. Available at: http://smi-web.stanford.edu/people/tcr/tcr-hsl-futures.html. Accessed January 14, 2003.

[52] Kronenfeld MR. Trends in academic health sciences libraries and their emergence as the "knowledge nexus" for their academic health centers. J Med Libr Assoc 2005;93(1): 32–9.

[53] Plutchak TS. Inept and satisfied, redux [editorial]. J Med Libr Assoc 2005;93(1):1–3.

[54] Harris MR. The librarian's roles in the systematic review process: a case study. J Med Libr Assoc 2005;93(1):81–7.

[55] McGowan J, Sampson M. Systematic reviews needs systematic searchers. J Med Libr Assoc 2005;93(1):74–80.

[56] Available at: http://www.health.library.mcgill.ca/course/Unit%207B%20Info%20Lit% 202004_files/frame.htm. Accessed June 8, 2005.

[57] Further information available at: http://www.dis.shef.ac.uk/literacy. Accessed December 19, 2005.

[58] SCONUL Advisory Committee on Information Literacy. Peters J. Learning outcomes and information literacy. The Higher Education Academy; 2004. Available at: http://www. sconul.ac.uk/pubs_stats/pubs/publications.html. Accessed December 19, 2005.

[59] Schilling K, Ginn DS, Mickelson P, et al. Integration of information-seeking skills and activities into a problem-based curriculum. Bull Med Libr Assoc 1995;83(2):176–83.

[60] Shershneva MB, Slotnick HB, Mejicano GC. Learning to use learning resources during medical school and residency. J Med Libr Assoc 2005;93(2):263–70.

[61] Vogel EW, Block KR, Wallingford KT. Finding the evidence: teaching medical residents to search MEDLINE. J Med Libr Assoc 2002;90(3):327–30.

[62] Palmer J. Future proofing the profession. SCONUL Focus 2004;33:55–60.

[63] Gallagher PE, compiler. Evidence-based medicine: a bibliography. Available at: http:// www.ebmny.org/ebmbib.html. Accessed October 31, 2005.

[64] Birch DW, Eady A, Robertson D, et al, for the Evidence-Based Surgery Working Group. Users' guide to the surgical literature: how to perform a literature search. Can J Surg 2003;46(2):136–41.

[65] Hong D, Randan VR, Goldsmith CH, et al, for the Evidence-Based Surgery Working Group. Users' guide to the surgical literature: how to use an article reporting population-based volume-outcome relationships in surgery. Can J Surg 2002;45(2):109–15.

[66] Birch DW, Goldsmith CH, Tandan V for the Evidence-Based Surgery Working Group. Users' guide to the surgical literature: self-audit and practice appraisal for surgeons. Can J Surg 2005;48(1):57–62.

[67] Centre for Evidence-Based Medicine. Searching for the best evidence in clinical journals. Available at: http://www.cebm.net/searching.asp. Accessed June 8, 2005.

[68] Netting the evidence. Available at: http://www.nettingtheevidence.org.uk. Accessed October 21, 2005.

[69] Toedter LJ, Thompson LL, Rohatgi C. Training surgeons to do evidence-based surgery: a collaborative approach. J Am Coll Surg 2004;199(2):293–9.

[70] Fingerhut A, Borie F, Dziri C. How to teach evidence-based surgery. World J Surg 2005; 29(5):592–5.

[71] Haines SJ, Nicholas JS. Teaching evidence-based medicine to surgical subspecialty residents. J Am Coll Surg 2003;197:285–9.

[72] Holst R, Funk CJ. State of the art of expert searching: results of a Medical Library Association survey. J Med Libr Assoc 2005;93(1):45–52.

[73] PICOmaker. Available at: http://www.library.ualberta.ca/pdazone/pico/index.cfm. Accessed October 31, 2005.

[74] Brice A, Muir Gray JA. What is the role of the librarian in 21st century healthcare? [guest editorial]. Health Inf Libr J 2004;21:81–3.

[75] Lynch, C. Check out the New Library [interview]. Ubiquity July 23–August 5, 2003;4(23). Available at: http://www.acm.org/ubiquity/interviews/pf/c_lynch_1.html. Accessed August 16, 2003.

[76] Marcum JW. Visions: the academic library in 2012. D-Lib Magazine May 2003;9(5). Available at: http://dlib.org/dlib/may03/marcum/05marcum.html. Accessed December 19, 2005.

[77] Simon JH. Planning the academic library of the 21st century: remarks of Jeanne Hurley Simon, Chairperson, US National Commission on Libraries and Information Science. Speech presented to University of Chicago Library Visiting Committee. Chicago, April 3, 1997. Available at: http://www.nclis.gov/about/speeches/simon/uchic.html. Accessed August 13, 2003.

ELSEVIER
SAUNDERS

Surg Clin N Am 86 (2006) 91–100

SURGICAL
CLINICS OF
NORTH AMERICA

Evidence-Based Surgery: Creating the Culture

Martin J.R. Lee, MA, MSc, FRCS

*University Hospitals, Coventry and Warwickshire National Health Service Trust,
Walsgrave Hospital, Clifford Bridge Road, Coventry CV2 2DX, England, UK*

The obligation of individual doctors to keep up to date and maintain their clinical skills is clearly identified by regulatory bodies. For example, in the United Kingdom, one of the duties of a doctor laid down by the General Medical Council (GMC) is to "keep your professional knowledge and skills up to date" [1], and in the Canadian Medical Education Directions for Specialists model of the Royal College of Physicians and Surgeons of Canada, being a "medical expert" links together other key roles of a doctor as a professional, a communicator, a scholar, a collaborator, a health advocate, and a manager [2].

From junior trainee to experienced consultant, how can we create a culture and environment that will support surgeons in these efforts, so that they can maintain and extend their knowledge base, keep their clinical practice up to date, and perform within accepted guidelines? To do so will not only improve surgeons' education and help protect them from litigation and professional failure, whatever the stage of their career, but will also benefit their patients. Indeed, such an approach is of importance as public expectations of health care rise and we move to an era of wider choice for patients and greater accountability for doctors, reflected in a renegotiation of the social compact between the medical profession, the public and governments [3].

The changing expectations of patients

Patients who have problems requiring surgery legitimately expect to be seen by surgeons who are experts—specialists in their fields rather than generalists—and to be offered treatment supported by an evidence base and governed by clinical guidelines. In addition, they may wish to be involved

---

E-mail address: martin.lee@uhcw.nhs.uk

doi:10.1016/j.suc.2005.10.006   *surgical.theclinics.com*

in exchanging views on clinical management before decisions are made. Increasingly, they attend clinics armed with detailed information about their conditions, and may ask some very searching questions. The rising use of the Internet for health information is well-documented. In 2001 a survey of United States households [4] found that 40% used the Internet to look for advice or information about health or health care, and in the same year a study of United Kingdom orthopedic outpatients found that 8% had obtained Internet information on their conditions, rising to 22% of those attending a regional tertiary referral clinic [5]. More recently, in primary care, 53% of patients had used the Web or e-mail in the previous year, 68% of these to search for health information [6].

Qualitative research suggests that, although use of the Internet can increase patients' knowledge about their health conditions, they may often be too overwhelmed or confused by the information available to make informed decisions. For example, American oncologists observed both positive and negative effects in the estimated one third of their patients who had used the Internet to obtain cancer information [7]. Their patients were noted to be simultaneously more hopeful, confused, anxious, and knowledgeable, and required on average 10 minutes longer for consultations.

Although some may view the extent of freely available information as a negative influence, challenging their medical authority and leading to inappropriate self-diagnosis (so-called "cyberchondria"), patients retain great faith in their doctors, and it is likely that the hype around Internet use by patients exceeds the reality. Nonetheless, we need to acknowledge that our patients and their families now have access to medical knowledge that is enabling them to be better-informed, and to take a greater part in making decisions about their care. In practice, this is reflected in organizational initiatives such as the United Kingdom National Health Service (NHS) "Choose and Book" program, in which patients are given "a greater opportunity to influence the way they are treated by the NHS" and will "be able to discuss their treatment options so that they experience a more personalized health service" [8].

There is undoubtedly a need for guidance through the mass of available knowledge, both for patients and health care professionals. How are surgeons to keep themselves ahead of this rising curve of publicly available information, creating a culture of continuous learning and updating in their institutions that can be absorbed by the whole of the multidisciplinary specialty team?

The need for better access to information for doctors

In the acute hospital setting, we need not only to provide better information support for patients, but also for doctors and the multiprofessional care team. Whatever is driving patients' concerns, be it information from the Internet, the media, or advice from family and friends, their doctors need to be able to respond authoritatively and promptly. Busy surgeons need readily available information to support their elective and emergency work on a 24-hour basis, and to achieve this a comprehensive and well-organized hospital intranet system, accessible at the point of care, is essential. Such systems should provide access to key portions of the patient record, such as investigation reports and correspondence, as well as links for professional sites, textbooks, guidelines, protocols, and literature searches.

Although hospital intranets have in many instances been dominated by administrative and performance data, greater benefits for patient care are likely to come from improving clinical functionality. Unfortunately, although systems and software have been put in place to allow this, the necessary education to get doctors, and surgeons in particular, using them has not always followed. Physical access and old, slow hardware can be a problem, particularly in busy clinical areas such as operating theaters where the available computer terminals are often in demand by other staff for administration and e-mails rather than for getting clinical information.

Handheld computers have been hailed as a solution to the challenge of the provision of point-of-care assistance. Such personal digital assistants can deliver a whole range of functions, including drug information, clinical guidelines, decision aids, patient tracking, clinical results, medical education, lecture notes, presentations, patient education, photographs, and diagrams. In practice, however, although some doctors are enthusiastic about using handheld computers to support their clinical work, these devices may not be the answer; concerns remain over reliability, security, and ease of use, and there is still a preference for paper [9].

Apart from being of benefit to undergraduate and postgraduate medical education, immediate online access to surgical textbooks, journals, and literature searches can support trainee doctors in the acute clinical situation. Examples of useful sites are the treatment guidelines available from the Royal College of Surgeons of Edinburgh Surgical Knowledge and Skills Web site (http://www.edu.rcsed.ac.uk/) and eMedicine (http://www.emedicine.com/). The United Kingdom National Electronic Library for Health (http://www.nelh.nhs.uk/) provides access via an Athens access management system password to a collection of over 1200 full-text journals, evidence bases, a guidelines finder, protocols, and a care pathways site, with links to Medline and PubMed. In addition to providing links to these sites, hospitals should also have easy access on their intranet to current locally adopted guidelines, and should ensure that there is a regulated process for update and review.

Surgeons' attitudes to information technology

Evidence from the United Kingdom would suggest that surgeons do not appear to have a very positive view of their hospital information systems. Doctors' perceptions of information technology (IT) systems were studied in a recent survey sent to all medical staff in NHS acute hospital trusts

[10,11]. It emerged that surgeons were the specialty group least likely to use IT systems, or to feel they could get the information they need about their patients from their hospital computer. Furthermore, surgeons felt less proficient than their colleagues in the use of these systems, with only half using NHS e-mail, and only a third believing that their trust IT system had improved patient care. Paradoxically, although a previous Audit Commission report had estimated that 25% of clinicians' time is spent collecting and using patient data [12], only two thirds of trusts had a system that allowed staff to access laboratory test results throughout the hospital. Doctors reported greater use of systems in which a higher proportion of hospital revenue was spent on information management and technology, and were more likely to become engaged in managing and developing IT when their hospitals had clinically integrated systems and offered training to new staff.

It is evident that if hospitals were to invest in and manage their information systems more effectively, then a significant burden on clinicians' time could be reduced, and clinical engagement improved. Regrettably, there is significant IT underinvestment in the NHS in comparison with other sectors of the economy and with health services in other comparable countries. It remains to be seen whether the introduction of a national program for information technology [13] to address the lack of central standards and incompatible systems will improve clinical IT functionality across the NHS. Involvement of clinicians and encouragement of medical use of systems is not only the remit of IT managers, but also an issue for medical and clinical directors locally, and professional associations nationally. Close involvement of clinicians in IT development is the key to realizing the benefits of systems, and internal performance management of hospital computer services should include monitoring staff acceptance of systems, and the attitudes of clinicians toward them.

It is difficult to put evidence-based surgery into practice without accurate and up-to-the-minute patient electronic records, capable of supporting multispecialty clinical communication and providing the information needed for effective handover of care. This is much needed in an era of regulated doctors' hours and shift working patterns, and along with IT, facilities for results alerts and decision support should have significant benefits for patient safety [14].

Educational support

Surgeons will be much better equipped to practice evidence-based surgery if they receive formal training in the skills needed to define precise clinical questions, and then access and critically appraise the relevant literature in search of an answer. Trainees should be encouraged to incorporate this attitude into their daily clinical activities, using for example the "PICO" approach to define the question: Patient's problem, Intervention under study, Comparative standard intervention, and Outcome variables of interest. This approach has been followed by the Dutch Society for Surgery, which has introduced an evidence-based surgery course in its surgical training program [15].

Lack of clinician time is frequently an issue, and one way in which this has been addressed is by introducing an expert librarian function into daily patient care. Such clinical librarian services have been developed with the aim of bringing health sciences library and literature searching expertise directly into the clinical scene [16]. As well as devoting time in the library to searching, collating, and producing information, the clinical librarian joins the multidisciplinary team at ward rounds, teaching sessions, and clinical conferences. This may overcome some difficulties that clinicians encounter when they attempt to incorporate the best current evidence from the literature into their patient care decisions. Perhaps of equal importance in the librarian role is the sharing and developing of these skills with the whole of the clinical team, as an educational experience for students, doctors in training, and also established consultants. Although clinical librarianship has become widely recognized and advocated, it has not been widely adopted, and further studies are required to confirm its value in comparison with other methods for supporting evidence-based health care in clinical settings [17].

Bringing together patient information and consent

Surgeons now have to spend more and more time in obtaining properly informed consent from patients for procedures. This whole process of consent has been the subject of increasing scrutiny in the NHS, with patients being encouraged to ask their surgeons for detailed information on treatment options, benefits, and risks, and how their outcomes compare locally and nationally. The surgeon is also expected to explain why an operation is necessary, what the risks are of doing nothing, and what the expected postoperative progress is; such as how patients will feel, when they are likely to get back to work, and what implications there are for their lifestyle, including effects on sport, exercise, diet, and personal and sexual relationships.

It is of particular importance to have clear guidance readily available that can be shared with patients on the supporting evidence for new treatments and techniques. In the United Kingdom, the National Institute for Health and Clinical Excellence (NICE; http://www.nice.org.uk/) provides a variety of guidance for a range of issues, including new drugs, interventional procedures, technology assessments, and clinical practice. Although it can be frustrating to wait for approval from NICE before embarking on a particular aspect of therapy, it is reassuring and in the best interests of patients to have a regulatory process, as long as innovation is not stifled and decisions are not made purely on grounds of financial expediency. Novel techniques need to be assessed, and the competence of surgeons in performing them evaluated. Local clinical governance arrangements should be in place to ensure that hospitals are aware when new procedures are being introduced, and are satisfied that their surgeons are trained in them and their patients properly informed. The NICE system for monitoring new procedures considers safety and efficacy, and produces drafts guidelines for use [18]. The success of this approach will depend on establishing comprehensive national databases and monitoring longer-term outcomes.

Because consent is a process in which the whole clinical team should be involved so that all these questions can be addressed and answered, the patients' need for information on elective surgery really begins in primary care when they see their general practitioners. In this context, systems such as PRODIGY (http://www.prodigy.nhs.uk/ClinicalGuidance/), a primary care-based source of evidence-based knowledge on managing common conditions and symptoms, can be particularly useful, with downloadable information leaflets for patients and links to many other sites.

Ultimately, however, responsibility rests with the operating surgeon to ensure that the patient has received sufficient information to make an informed judgment about the proposed treatment before proceeding. Such a process demands not only the need for up-to-date and accurate information about best evidence-based treatment, but also highlights that surgeons should know their individual and unit results, and how they compare with national and international standards. Ensuring that surgeons have, own, and can trust this information is another crucial step in establishing the local culture for evidence-based practice.

The importance of knowing your results

In a world in which patients expect their surgeons to be experts, it is important to have accurate information on outcomes. Awareness of these outcomes is valuable to the surgeon as well as the patient, for how are we to improve our standards of care unless we take account of the results of our interventions?

Public access to individual surgeon performance in the United Kingdom has been hotly debated, particularly in the light of requests for data following the implementation of freedom of information legislation. A recommendation of the inquiry into pediatric cardiac surgery deaths at the Bristol Royal Infirmary was that patients should be able to see information about the results of surgeons operating in hospitals [19]. The Society of Cardiothoracic Surgeons of Great Britain and Ireland therefore published a study in 2004 of activity and performance of all consultants undertaking adult cardiac surgery in the United Kingdom [20]. The Freedom of Information Act, which has now become law in England and Wales, gives a general right of access to all types of recorded information held by public authorities. Under the Act it is inevitable that individual surgeon data will come into the public domain, and some individual hospitals are already responding by putting results on the Internet. It is essential that such publicity should not ultimately disadvantage patients by engendering a culture in which surgeons anxious to obtain good overall mortality results turn down the higher risk patients, who may have the most to gain from successful surgery. Other risks that must be borne in mind are those of discounting patient preferences, overlooking clinical judgment, and aiming to hit "target rates" for interventions when the procedure may be inappropriate for that patient. Thus it is crucial that surgeons are intimately involved in the process of standard setting and data collection, and in defining appropriate measures for risk stratification. This involvement in standard setting should also highlight the need to be continually seeking the evidence to support clinical interventions; a natural step beyond this is to participate in development of and recruitment to high-quality studies that will guide future clinical care.

It is also vital that surgeons should understand and influence the motives behind public reporting of information. Quality information should allow patients, referring doctors, and health care purchasers to choose high-quality surgeons. It should also motivate surgeons to strive for high standards, and through a peer review process to identify and assist each other with areas for improvement. The benefits of such a process have been well-demonstrated in the NHS breast screening program [21], in which a national peer review process performed for more than a decade has brought about major improvements in data quality, and significantly raised standards in diagnosis and treatment for women with breast cancer.

"Dr Foster" is an independent organization that provides research, analysis and communication products to health care providers in the United Kingdom (http://www.drfoster.co.uk/hp/index.asp). Through links with the NHS and Department of Health, Dr Foster's professed aim is to add value in policy areas such as clinical information, patient choice, and public health. The site developers have set up a Web-based system for acute hospitals that records standard hospital episode data down to the individual consultant level. This is analyzed to provide information on mortality, length of stay, and other parameters in an online "clinical monitoring and benchmarking service" that compares, specialty by specialty, current performance with peer groups nationally, automatically alerting managers and senior clinicians to significant variation from expected performance. Data are standardized by individual patients in an effort to achieve comparability between trusts, and are based on routine hospital episode statistics. Hospitals and departments can choose their own peer groups, which gives the opportunity for making realistic comparisons of practices and outcomes. As well as entering the public domain and influencing patient referrals, the analysis may be used to identify areas of good clinical practice, or where there are concerns that need to be addressed, down even to the level of individual consultant performance.

Clinical governance: organization versus freedom?

Modern acute hospitals contain many specialties and departments and employ hundreds of consultants. It is a challenge to achieve consistent standards of care in this situation against a background of many conflicting demands: personalized versus regulated care, emergency versus elective access, vagaries of resource provision, and service commissioning. This is the essence of a current debate on the effectiveness of clinical governance. As Degeling and colleagues [22] point out, recognizing that clinicians are at the core of clinical work is central to re-establishing the "responsible autonomy" that is the foundation of the performance and organization of clinical work. They raise crucial questions that need to be asked: Are we doing the right things? Are we doing the things right? Are we keeping up with new developments? And what are we doing to extend our capacity to undertake clinical work in these areas?

Top-down management, driven by the need to achieve performance targets, often disengages clinicians, who view clinical governance as a management-driven exercise that has increased administrative activity to the detriment of patient care. To reverse this trend, clinicians and managers need to understand the links between clinical care and resource, to achieve a balance between clinical autonomy and accountability, to support a systematic approach to clinical work, and to accept the power-sharing implications of better-integrated approaches to clinical work and its evaluation.

Clinical management structures are important in establishing a coherent and effective team approach in which evidence-based care can be embedded. Management structures should provide a clinical environment that encourages and facilitates clinical supervision, professional advice and support, continuing professional development and update, and professional accountability and audit. The clinical management team should also develop support for teaching and training, research and development, strategy and business planning, career development, and clinical governance issues, including competence. The needs of accredited specialists and trainees are similar, in that there should be clearly stated processes for mentoring and appraisal, with identified time in the weekly timetable, and administrative and technological support.

Integrated care pathways will allow large amounts of elective and emergency care to be systematized, and the clinical governance support in surgical departments should then enable their high-volume work to be systematically studied and improved, integrating financial control, service performance, and clinical quality. Only by such close working of clinical teams and managers can we create a culture in which the evidence base that supports care is continuously incorporated in the model of care, with appropriate resource allocation.

How do we find the time to do all this?

Time is an issue, and although the new consultant contract in the United Kingdom recognizes the need for "supporting professional activities," on average only 10 hours per week are allotted to cover activities that include provision of training and medical education, continuing professional development, formal teaching, clinical audit, job planning, appraisal, research, clinical management, and local clinical governance activities. For consultants, a compounding effect has been the reduction in availability of resident trainees resulting from implementation of working time regulations. In turn, the trainees themselves have reduced opportunities for clinical and operative experience and other educational activities. All this makes it of even greater importance that efficient IT systems reduce wastage of clinician time on unnecessary administrative tasks, and that information is readily available to support evidence-based care in clinical settings. One could argue that to cope in today's world, the surgeon must be equally at home with the computer as with the scalpel or the laparoscope.

Summary

At a time when the relationship between patients and their doctors is under scrutiny, and what constitutes medical professionalism is being re-evaluated, it is essential that we establish in our institutions a culture that supports one of the key elements of professionalism, namely knowledge. The expectation for individuals and clinical teams to be keeping up to date must be embedded, and supported by providing the equipment and facilities to do so. This will allow a shared agenda between managers and surgeons in providing high-quality care for patients.

References

[1] Good medical practice. General Medical Council 2002. Available at http://www.gmc-uk. org/guidance/library/GMP.pdf. Accessed June 12, 2005.
[2] The CanMEDS Project overview. The Royal College of Physicians of Surgeons of Canada. Available at: http://rcpsc.medical.org/canmeds/index.php. Accessed June 12, 2005.
[3] On being a doctor. In: Rosen R, Dewar S, editors. Redefining medical professionalism for better patient care. Kings Fund Publications; 2004.
[4] Baker L, Wagner TH, Singer S, et al. Use of the Internet and e-mail for health care information: results from a national survey. JAMA 2003;289:2400–6.
[5] Wright JED, Brown RR, Chadwick C, et al. The use of the Internet by orthopaedic outpatients. J Bone Joint Surg Br 2001;83-B:1096–7.
[6] Dickerson S, Reinhart AM, Feeley TH, et al. Patient Internet use for health information at three urban primary care clinics. J Am Med Inform Assoc 2004;11:499–504.
[7] Helft PR, Hlubocky F, Daugherty CK. American oncologists' views of Internet use by cancer patients: a mail survey of American Society of Clinical Oncology members. J Clin Oncol 2003;21:942–7.
[8] Choose & book patient's choice of hospital and booked appointment: policy framework for choice and booking at the point of referral. Department of Health. August 2004. www.dh. gov.uk/assetRoot/04/08/83/52/04088352.pdf. Accessed May 15, 2005.
[9] McAlearney AS, Schweikhart SB, Medow MA. Doctors' experience with handheld computers in clinical practice: qualitative study. BMJ 2004;328:1162.
[10] Information and records guidance. Available at: http://www.healthcarecommission. org.uk./informationforserviceproviders/guidanceforNHS/guidance/fs/en?CONTENTid = 4002328&CHK = Qb%2Bhjg. Accessed May 29, 2005.

[11] Smith D, Bailey J, Boyce J. Doctors' perceptions of the IT systems in their NHS acute and specialist trusts. Br J Healthcare Comput Info Manage 2004;21(8):16–9.

[12] Audit Commission. For your information: a study of information management and systems in the acute hospital. London: HMSO; 1995.

[13] Department of Health; June 2002. Delivering 21st century IT support for the NHS—national strategic programme. Available at: http://www.dh.gov.uk/assetRoot/04/06/71/12/04067112.pdf. Accessed May 29, 2005.

[14] Ubbink DT, Legemate DA. Evidence-based surgery. Br J Surg 2004;91:1091–2.

[15] Bates DW. Using information technology to improve surgical safety. Br J Surg 2004;91:939–40.

[16] Weightman AL, Williamson J. The value and impact of information provided through library services for patient care: a systematic review. Health Info Libr J 2005;22(1):4–25.

[17] Wagner KC, Byrd GD. Evaluating the effectiveness of clinical medical librarian programs: a systematic review of the literature. J Med Libr Assoc 2004;92(1):14–33.

[18] Campbell WR, Barnett DB. The governance of Innovation. Br J Surg 2004;91:1536–7.

[19] Learning from Bristol. The report of the public inquiry into children's heart surgery at the Bristol Royal Infirmary 1984–1995. Available at: http://www.bristol-inquiry.org.uk/final_report/the_report/pdf. Accessed June 17, 2005.

[20] Keogh BE, Kinsman R. Fifth national adult cardiac surgical database report 2003. Henley on Thames (UK): Dendrite Clinical Systems; 2004.

[21] Changing Lives. NHS breast screening programme annual review 2004. NHS cancer screening programmes. Available at: http://www.cancerscreening.nhs.uk/breastscreen/publications/nhsbsp-annualreview2004.pdf. Accessed June 17, 2005.

[22] Degeling PJ, Maxwell S, Iedema R, et al. Making clinical governance work. BMJ 2004;329:679–81.

ELSEVIER
SAUNDERS

SURGICAL
CLINICS OF
NORTH AMERICA

Surg Clin N Am 86 (2006) 101–114

Systematic Reviews of Surgical Interventions

Martin Burton, MA, DM[a],*, Mike Clarke, MA, DPhil[b]

[a]*Department of Otolaryngology-Head and Neck Surgery, University of Oxford,
The Radcliffe Infirmary, Oxford OX2 6HE, England, UK*
[b]*United Kingdom Cochrane Centre, Middle Way, Summertown,
Oxford OX2 7LG, England, UK*

All physicians are familiar with the type of general review articles found in many medical journals. Systematic reviews are different. They apply a strict, scientific methodology to the reviewing process to produce a review that is comprehensive, reliable, and as free from bias as possible. As a result, systematic reviews occupy the highest position in the "levels of evidence" tables associated with the practice of evidence-based health care.

Systematic reviews are not limited to reviews of randomized trials of the effects of treatments, but can and do exist for other types of study also. Systematic reviews can be done for topics such as causes of disease, prognosis and prognostic factors, diagnostic test accuracy, and genetics. The appropriate study design to include in a review depends on the question to be answered; however, the well-done systematic review should always be at the top of the hierarchy, because it brings together all the relevant research and does not selectively focus only on research with a particular result. In this article, the authors discuss how systematic reviews can help to answer questions about the relative effects of treatments. As such, focus is on reviews of randomized trials and the contribution that these make to evidence based health care.

Evidence-based medicine (EBM) has been defined as the conscientious, explicit, and judicious use of current best evidence in making decisions about the care of individual patients [1]. Although this term is widely used, it is also widely misused, and poorly understood. For the present, the key phrase is "current best evidence." In recent years there has been an explosion in the quantity of published medical information. The amount

---

* Corresponding author.
E-mail address: mburton@cochrane-ent.org (M. Burton).

of information available in journals, books, magazines, and the media in general was overwhelming a decade ago. The arrival of the Internet, with the enormous quantity of information it now contains and the ease with which vast amounts of material can be found, has added considerably to this burden. Some of the information available is of high quality and is reliable enough for decision making; unfortunately, much of what is available is of poor quality.

As a consequence, keeping up to date—once possible simply by reading the national surgical journals on a regular basis and attending a few meetings—is now much more difficult. The conscientious surgical practitioner has to be able to search out the evidence relating to his or her clinical query, appraise its quality, and then synthesize the results. The skills needed to do this successfully need to be learned and practiced, and this training process should be undertaken with the same diligence and perseverance applied to the acquisition of those manual skills required of the competent surgeon.

Fortunately, for many busy practitioners, an increasing number of systematic reviews now exist in which other researchers have already done much of this work. Later in this article, the authors discuss The Cochrane Collaboration and the contribution it and its members have made to helping people find, understand, and use reliable evidence quickly. Even if one finds a systematic review done by someone else, however, it still needs to be appraised to assess its quality and its relevance to the question at hand. Thus all practitioners, not just those who want to do a review, need to be familiar with the process and the steps needed to reduce bias. This article sets out this process.

Systematic reviews aim to locate, appraise, and synthesize evidence from scientific studies. To ensure that they are comprehensive, are least likely to be prone to bias, and to ensure their reliability, they adhere to a strict scientific design.

Developing a focused clinical question

At the outset, the reviewer formulates a clearly focused clinical question. This may be a question about therapy, diagnosis, prevention, or harm. The example given here is a question relating to a therapeutic intervention, but the reviewing process is similar when applied to other types of questions. Whatever its nature, the question must focus on the decisions faced by patients and practitioners.

An example might be: "Do perioperative antibiotics help prevent postoperative wound infections in patients undergoing appendicectomy?"

This has the standard three-part structure often found in well thought-out clinical questions. That is: (1) how effective is A, (2) for the management of B, (3) in patients who have C? It has a meaningful outcome (the prevention of wound infection) that is relevant to both the patient and doctor, and it is clearly focused. A less well-focused question might be: "Do antibiotics help prevent postoperative infections of any sort in surgical patients?"—much too broad. At the other extreme, questions that are too narrow in focus may turn out to be impossible (and irrelevant) to answer: "Does penicillin help prevent postoperative wound infections in young children who have complicated appendicitis?" The key components to the focused question in this example are

- The types of patients here, all patients, both children and adults, undergoing appendicectomy.
- The types of interventions and comparators here we are looking at any antibiotic regime versus no antibiotic, probably a placebo. An alternative review might look at direct comparisons of different antibiotic regimes.
- The types of outcomes we have specified wound infections, but will have to decide how specific we want to be about the diagnosis of these infections. For example, we need to decide if we are going to look for studies that insist on a microbiological diagnosis as opposed to a clinical one.

We then also need to consider the types of study design we are going to look for. Because randomized controlled trials (RCTs) are the least biased design for assessing the relative effects of interventions, many systematic reviews of treatment determine at the outset that they will only include RCTs. Some reviews, however, do include other types of study, but they need to be cautious about the potential for bias in these studies—biases that might lead to misleading conclusions about the true differences between the interventions in the review.

The quality criteria that are going to be applied to the RCTs that are found must also be considered. Just because an RCT is published in a reputable medical journal, it does not necessarily mean that the trial will be of high quality. Before undertaking a systematic review, it is necessary to state which features of a trial one believes are associated with high-quality studies (and therefore increased reliability and validity of the results). There is good evidence available on which features to investigate to allow this to be done.

Identifying relevant studies

Another important part of the process of undertaking a systematic review is trying to find all those RCTs that address the question of interest. Ideally one would find all those trials that have been published and all those unpublished. This is important because publication bias is well-recognized—a trial is more likely to get published if it has a positive result. There is therefore a danger that bringing together the results only of published trials will skew the results in favor of demonstrating a positive treatment effect, when in reality, had all trials been combined, no effect would have been demonstrated.

A second important bias to be avoided is language bias; there is no good a priori reason why a study published in a non-English language journal should be less relevant or of poorer quality than one published in a leading United Kingdom or North American journal. Clearly there may be difficulties in finding non-English language studies (of which more below), not to mention difficulty in translation. But these are not insurmountable, and international organizations that produce and publish high quality systematic reviews, such as The Cochrane Collaboration, are able to use the multinational, multilingual membership base as a tool for identifying and translating such studies.

Several methods should be used to identify the appropriate RCTs. Sensitive search strategies for the retrieval of RCTs have been developed for use with MEDLINE, EMBASE, and other electronic databases. The Cochrane Central Register of Controlled Trials (CENTRAL), published in the Cochrane Library, contains the product of such searches as well as the extensive searching of journals and conference proceedings that is ongoing within The Cochrane Collaboration [2]. In addition, CENTRAL includes studies that have been published in languages other than English, as well as records for ongoing and unpublished studies. As a result, CENTRAL is one of the best sources for reports of RCTs, and is easily searchable.

When searching any database, be it CENTRAL or the electronic bibliographic databases dedicated to the health care literature in general, it is important that the correct search terms are used to identify trials addressing the topic in question. It is helpful to elicit the assistance of an information specialist, because this process is not always as intuitive and simple as many physicians might believe at first. For example, searching using the term "appendectomy" will miss reports using the British spelling "appendicectomy," and those that simply mentioned the "removal of the appendix."

As well as searching CENTRAL and the other databases, the search for studies should include examination of the reference lists within the identified studies. One can also consider searching journals, because the indexing process used by MEDLINE and the like has not always identified RCTs in the older paper-based publications, and many journals are not indexed in databases that are readily accessible. As mentioned above, a coordinated approach to the searching of journals is being organized by The Cochrane Collaboration to avoid duplication of effort. Details of the journals that have been and are being hand-searched are available from The Cochrane Collaboration Web site (www.cochrane.org), and reports of RCTs identified are included in CENTRAL. Reviewers should also check conference proceedings and abstracts that might be particularly relevant. Many studies (especially those with negative results) are presented at meetings but get no further [3]. If abstracts reporting results of these studies can be identified, the authors can be contacted and further details of the trial obtained. It is also important to consider writing directly to experts in the chosen field to see if they are aware of any studies that have not been identified.

Sifting and appraising initial search results

The result of a comprehensive search is likely to be a set of titles and abstracts, some, but not all, of which will address the topic under evaluation. Usually, reading the titles and abstracts will allow some studies to be discarded as inappropriate for further evaluation, leaving a smaller set to be analyzed further. This first step is best done by more than one person [4]. After it has been completed, it becomes necessary to retrieve the original publications and begin the process of critical appraisal.

There are two steps in the process of critically appraising the individual studies, which can be considered as questions.

Is the study applicable to this systematic review?

Does it evaluate the intervention in question in the types of patient in question? Are the outcomes evaluated in the study those of interest? It is important to note at the outset of the systematic reviewing process that reviewers should state which outcome measures are of primary and secondary interest. Usually these will be things of direct relevance to patients and practitioners. Although it is always possible that the reviewer will overlook an important outcome, this is unlikely if sufficient care and attention has been paid at the beginning. It is more likely that a study will be identified that looks at an outcome not deemed important by the reviewers. In the example above, an RCT of perioperative antibiotics in patients undergoing appendicectomy might have used as its only outcome measure blood levels of an inflammatory mediator. In this type of case, the degree to which the measured variable can be considered an adequate surrogate measure for the outcome in question is important. In this example, this study would probably be excluded from the systematic review on the grounds that the outcome measure used was not appropriate; however, it might be worth contacting the authors to see if they did collect any outcomes that might be of relevance to the review.

At the end of this process, another subset of studies will have been excluded from the review.

What is the validity of the individual study?

In essence, is this a good or a bad study? Has the study been designed and conducted in such a way that bias has been reduced to the minimum? Specific biases include selection bias, performance bias, attrition bias, and detection bias. Good RCTs are designed to avoid these.

Briefly, "selection bias" occurs if there are systematic differences between the groups within a trial that might affect the prognosis or responsiveness to treatment of the patients in one of the groups. This is best prevented by randomization of large enough numbers of patients to each group, because this will both reduce the biases and the effects of chance. The allocation of patients to one group or the other should be concealed from the participants in the trial and the providers of care. This ensures that a preference for one of the treatments will not bias the entry into that group. It is the best way to minimize differences in confounding variables between the groups, and is the reason why reviews of the effects of interventions need to focus on randomized trials.

A decision to enter the patient into the trial should be made before the process of randomization, and those entering the patient should be unaware of the group to which the patient will be allocated. Good methods of randomization include remote randomization by telephone, or the use of sequentially numbered, sealed, opaque envelopes. The use of alternation, hospital numbers, birth date, day of entry into trial, and the like are not satisfactory methods because they are not always random and are open to manipulation. The sequence of patients can be changed to subvert the alternation process, and knowing which treatment a patient will receive might affect the decision on whether or not he takes part in the study.

"Performance bias" refers to the presence of differences in the care provided to the groups of patient other than the intervention being evaluated. This can be prevented by blinding care providers and participants, and standardizing the care protocol. In the review in our example, this might be achieved through the use of a placebo.

"Attrition bias" refers to any systematic differences between the groups in the pattern of withdrawal from the study (for example, dropouts because of side-effects, participants who failed to comply with their treatment, or those who crossed over into the other arm of a trial). In the latter case, in surgical trials, this may include patients randomized to the nonsurgical arm who actually receive surgery. The most appropriate measure to overcome this problem is the use of a so-called "intention-to-treat" analysis, in which all patients randomized are analyzed within the group to which they were allocated.

Finally, if there are systematic differences in how the outcomes are assessed between the groups, "detection bias" can occur. This is minimized by blinding the participants and outcome assessors. Again, in the review in the example above, the use of a placebo might help to achieve this.

Clearly, in surgical trials, it is much more difficult to avoid some of these biases. The cry is often heard "It's impossible to blind in surgical trials, because the surgeon always knows what operation she is doing." The truth of the second half of this sentence is self-evident, but the first statement is not true at all. The patient, the practitioner enrolling the patient in the trial, those providing postoperative care, and certainly those assessing the outcomes can, in many circumstances, be blinded as to the specific intervention in a study. This is especially the case when surgical procedure A is compared with procedure B. Even in some trials of surgical intervention versus nonsurgical treatment, those assessing outcome can be blinded as to whether or not a participant received the intervention.

Summarizing and using assessments of validity

Having answered these questions, there are two ways in which the validity of a study can be used by the reviewer (who will have stated a priori which method will be used). The first method is to only include papers with low risk of bias in the review. This is one option, and might be appropriate when a large number of trials have been identified. Only those trials designed and conducted to the very highest standards are included in the final analysis.

The second method is to summarize the risks of bias using a simple grading scale. For example, consider the specific biases and relate these to the design and conduct of the individual studies, and then categorize the studies using this scale

Grade A = low risk of bias
Grade B = medium risk
Grade C = high risk of bias.

Having done this, there are several options available for incorporating the grades into the reviewing process.

The grading system can be used to include or exclude studies from the review. For example, include A and B, exclude C. Alternatively, all grades of studies can be included in the review, and the grading may allow the reviewer to explain differences in the results when studies are compared.

More formally, the grades can be used as the basis for a sensitivity analysis. For example, imagine that the results of nine studies (three grade A, three grade B and three grade C) had been combined, and that the results showed that the treatment in question was effective. A sensitivity analysis would then assess how dependent this result was on the inclusion of the poorer quality studies. If the six studies graded B & C were excluded but the result remained the same, one could be confident about its veracity. If this exclusion resulted in a change, however—if the treatment was not effective when one looked simply at the grade A studies—this would be significant. The demonstration of effectiveness of the treatment being critically dependant on the inclusion of poorer quality studies clearly calls into question to certainty of that result.

The grades can also be used as "weights" in statistical analysis. Many, but not all, systematic reviews include a meta-analysis. The weight given to a particular study in that analysis usually depends on the number of participants in the trial; however, an alternative or supplementary approach is to use the grade of the study as one of the weighting factors.

Dealing with the included studies

Having been through the process of identifying and appraising individual studies, the reviewer will now know how many could be incorporated into the systematic review, and must decide whether or not the results of the studies can be mathematically combined. Thus far there has been little mention of statistics and meta-analysis. It is axiomatic that statistical methods for combining the results of studies provide a powerful tool for deriving potentially important and useful conclusions from data. Equally, they provide a means by which errors of interpretation can be made. Having said that, it may be neither possible nor sensible to combine data sets from individual studies. Each study may have measured outcomes in such a different way that the results cannot be combined. For example, two studies examining the effectiveness of a perioperative intervention on postoperative pain control may have measured postoperative pain in different ways. One may use pain scores based on visual analog scales, and the other may use the need for supplemental postoperative analgesia. Both are equally valid ways to measure pain, but the specific results cannot easily be mathematically combined.

Sometimes the outcome measures used by the studies are different, but another dichotomous variable can be calculated from these data. For example, if a scoring system has been used to measure patients' symptoms before and after an intervention or placebo, it may be possible to compute the "proportion of patients improved" in each case. Even if a number of studies have used different scoring systems, this proportion may be calculable for each study, and as a result, the study results can be combined.

There are several benefits of doing a meta-analysis if it is proper so to do. First, to obtain a more precise estimate of the treatment effect and to be more certain about the size of the effect. Second, there is more statistical power to detect small effects that may be clinically significant. Finally, meta-analysis allows evaluation of the generalizability of the results. It cannot be emphasized enough, however, that to do a meta-analysis when there are no relevant, valid data, or when it does not make sense, is inappropriate. Furthermore, one of the important decisions that a reviewer has to make is whether the trials are not so dissimilar that an average of their results would be meaningless. This is done by considering whether there is excessive heterogeneity in the design of the studies (including the interventions and participants studied and the outcomes measured), and statistical tests are also available to assess whether the results of a series of trials might differ from each other by more than chance [5].

Statistical methods

There are a variety of statistical variables and methods used in systematic reviews and meta-analyses, and these will not be discussed further here; however, the fundamental principle is that participants in one trial are never directly compared with those from another trial. A statistical result is calculated for each trial independently, and then these statistics are combined [6].

The Cochrane Collaboration

As we have discussed already, systematic reviews are vital to the interpretation of research evidence, to its placing in context, and to its use in evidence-based decision-making. These reviews need to be kept up-to-date because the research base on which they are built rarely stands still. The Cochrane Collaboration is the largest organization in the world engaged in the production and maintenance of systematic reviews. It has received worldwide support in its efforts to make systematic reviews accessible to people making decisions about health care. Cochrane reviews bring together the relevant research findings on a particular topic, synthesize this evidence, and then present it in a standard, structured way. One of their most important attributes is that they are periodically updated to take account of new studies and other new information, to help people be confident that the systematic reviews are sufficiently current to be useful in making decisions about health care.

The Cochrane Collaboration was established in 1993, founded on ideas and ideals that stem from earlier times. In October 1992, Iain Chalmers, Kay Dickersin, and Thomas Chalmers began an editorial in the BMJ [7] with words from the British epidemiologist, Archie Cochrane, published in 1972:

> It is surely a great criticism of our profession that we have not organized a critical summary, by specialty or subspecialty, updated periodically, of all relevant randomized controlled trial [8].

This editorial was published at the time of the opening of the first Cochrane Center in Oxford, England. A year after this Centre opened, the first Cochrane Colloquium was held, bringing together 77 people from 19 countries, and they established The Cochrane Collaboration as an international organization. There are now eleven further Cochrane Centers, in Australia, Brazil, Canada, China, Denmark, Germany, Holland, Italy, South Africa, Spain, and the United States; with branches of these centers in several other countries.

There are currently more than 13,000 people contributing to the work of the Cochrane Collaboration from almost 100 countries, and this involvement continues to grow. The number of people involved has increased by 10% to 20% year on year for each of the 6 years to 2005.

The Cochrane Collaboration has ten guiding principles:

1. Collaboration, by internally and externally fostering good communications, open decision-making, and teamwork
2. Building on the enthusiasm of individuals, by involving and supporting people of different skills and backgrounds
3. Avoiding duplication, by good management and coordination, to maximize economy of effort
4. Minimizing bias, through a variety of approaches such as scientific rigor, ensuring broad participation, and avoiding conflicts of interest

5. Keeping up to date, by a commitment to ensure that Cochrane Reviews are maintained through identification and incorporation of new evidence
6. Striving for relevance, by promoting the assessment of health care interventions using outcomes that matter to people making choices in health care
7. Promoting access, by wide dissemination of the outputs of The Cochrane Collaboration, taking advantage of strategic alliances, and by promoting appropriate prices, content, and media to meet the needs of users worldwide
8. Ensuring quality by being open and responsive to criticism, applying advances in methodology, and developing systems for quality improvement
9. Continuity, by ensuring that responsibility for reviews, editorial processes, and key functions is maintained and renewed
10. Enabling wide participation in the work of The Cochrane Collaboration by reducing barriers to contributing and by encouraging diversity.

Preparation, maintenance, and accessibility of Cochrane reviews

The work of preparing and maintaining Cochrane reviews is done by the authors of Cochrane reviews working with one of 50 Cochrane Collaborative review groups, which collectively provide a home for reviews in all aspects of health care interventions. These groups are responsible for particular areas of health care, usually based around a particular condition or state of health. For example, there is a Breast Cancer Group with an editorial base in Sydney, Australia and a Pregnancy and Childbirth Group based in Liverpool, England. There are also groups in particular specialties such as ear, nose and throat (Oxford, United Kingdom) and anesthesia (Copenhagen, Denmark). The Cochrane Collaborative review groups organize the refereeing of the drafts for protocols for Cochrane reviews (which set out how the review will be done), and for the reviews themselves. The editorial teams in these groups have the ultimate decision on whether or not a Cochrane review should be published. But, unlike editors in more traditional health care journals, their role is, in part, to help the authors of Cochrane reviews ensure that their review becomes good enough to be published; the decision that a Cochrane review will be published depends on its quality, not its findings. The main motivation for most authors of Cochrane reviews is a desire to answer reliably a question about the relative effects of interventions for people who have particular conditions—very few of them receive any direct payment for this work.

The Collaborative review groups are based around the world, and some have editorial bases in more than one country. There are also Cochrane methods groups, with expertise in relevant areas of methodology; fields, or networks, with broad areas of interest and expertise spanning the scope of many review groups; and a consumer network helping to promote the interests of users of health care. The Cochrane Collaboration Steering Group, containing elected members from these different types of entity and Cochrane centers, is responsible for setting collaboration-wide policy and, by working with the entities, the implementation of the Collaboration's strategic plan.

As noted above, The Cochrane Collaboration grew rapidly through its first decade in terms of the number of people involved. Its output has also grown quickly. Cochrane reviews are published in full in The Cochrane Database of Systematic Reviews (CDSR), and the first issue of this in early 1995 contained 36 Cochrane reviews. A decade later there were nearly 2500, with published protocols for 1600 more. Various milestones have been passed along the way. There were 500 Cochrane reviews in 1999, and the one thousandth appeared in 2001, with 2000 published by April 2004. Hundreds of newly completed reviews and protocols are added each year, and a few hundred existing reviews are updated so substantively that they can be considered to be the equivalent of new reviews.

The Cochrane Database of Systematic Reviews is available on the Internet and on CD-ROM as part of The Cochrane Library. This is published by John Wiley and Sons Ltd. and is available on a subscription basis. The establishment of national contracts means that The Cochrane Library is currently free at the point of use to everyone in the United Kingdom and Ireland, as well as in Australia, Denmark, Finland, Norway, and South Africa.

The output of The Cochrane Collaboration also includes the Cochrane Central Register of Controlled Trials (CENTRAL), the Cochrane Database of Methodology Reviews, and the Cochrane Methodology Register. All of which are unique resources. In 1993, when the Collaboration was established, fewer than 20,000 reports of randomized trials could be found easily in MEDLINE, and one of the main tasks facing the Collaboration was the need to identify and make accessible information on reports of trials that might be suitable for inclusion in Cochrane reviews. It has done this through extensive programs of the hand searching of journals (in which a journal is checked from cover to cover to look for relevant reports) and of electronic searching of bibliographic databases such as MEDLINE and EMBASE. Suitable records are then added to CENTRAL, with coordination by the US Cochrane Centre in Rhode Island [2]. By 2004, CENTRAL contained records for more than 400,000 reports of randomized (or possibly randomized) trials, many of which are not included in any other electronic database. The Cochrane Database of Methodology Reviews contains the full text for Cochrane methodology reviews, which are systematic reviews of issues relevant to the conduct of reviews of health care interventions or evaluations of health care more generally. In 2005, there are 11 full Cochrane methodology reviews and published protocols for 9 more. The Cochrane Methodology Register, to a large extent, provides the raw material for the Cochrane methodology reviews. It contains more than 7000 records relating to the methodology of systematic reviews and other types of evaluation of health care, including many records relevant to trials and other evaluations of surgery.

Over the next few years, The Cochrane Collaboration will strive to ensure that its work is sustainable. Even with more than 4000 Cochrane reviews already underway, and results available from 2000 of these, there is still a large amount of work to be done. It has been estimated that approximately 10,000 systematic reviews are needed to cover all health care interventions that have already been investigated in controlled trials [9], and such reviews would need to be assessed and, if necessary, updated at the rate of 5000 per year. If the growth in The Cochrane Collaboration continues at the pace of the last few years, this target will be reached within the coming 10 years; however, this will require continuing and evolving partnership and collaboration. The Cochrane Collaboration will need to continue to attract and support the wide variety of people who contribute to its work. It will also need to work together with funders and with providers of health care to ensure that the resources needed for the work grow, and that the output of the work is accessible to people making decisions about health care around the world [10].

Systematic reviews of surgical interventions: challenges and examples

The Cochrane Database of Systematic Reviews now contains many examples of systematic reviews of surgical interventions or of issues relevant to surgery. Such reviews might not be as straightforward as reviews of a homogenous series of randomized trials containing similar participants, allocated to receive a drug at a particular dose versus a matching placebo, with the effects assessed using an unequivocal endpoint such as death; however, reviews that are this straightforward are rare.

Systematic reviews of surgical interventions do present particular challenges, just as randomized trials of these interventions can be challenging. Whenever a person is a key component of the intervention, as is the case with surgical skill, there may be a learning curve; or the surgeon might be much more proficient at one of the interventions. Trial designs, such as randomizing patients to the operator rather than the operation, have been suggested and would be amenable to systematic reviews [11]. The difficulties of "blinding" were mentioned above, but as discussed, mechanisms can be put in place to ensure that the person assessing outcomes does not know what intervention a patient was allocated to. Identical wound dressings can just as easily cover a short incision as the smaller hole used for a laparascopic incision in gallbladder removal.

And even if the randomized trials are not thought to exist for some important surgical questions, a systematic review will still prove beneficial by confirming this lack of evidence, drawing attention to the gaps, and highlighting how the necessary research might be done. All new research should be preceded by a systematic review to ensure that the necessary research has not already been done and to facilitate the design of the most appropriate and feasible trial [12].

Just to provide some flavor of systematic reviews of surgical interventions that now exist, the authors had a browse in The Cochrane Database of Systematic Reviews. It was not very difficult to find that reviews have been done of preoperative management (bowel preparation before colorectal surgery [13]), different surgical techniques (for treating distal radial fractures [14]), surgery versus other invasive procedures (neurosurgical clipping versus endovascular coiling for subarachnoid hemorrhage [15]); and postoperative wound management (tap water versus other ways to cleanse wounds [16]).

Systematic reviews relevant to surgery are no less relevant than systematic reviews in other areas of health care. They should be a prerequisite of any new research, a key component in decision making, and an opportunity for all surgical practitioners to get involved in the conduct and interpretation of research.

References

[1] Sackett DL, Rosenberg WMC, Gray JAM, et al. Evidence-based medicine: what it is and what it isn't. BMJ 1996;312:71–2.

[2] Dickersin K, Manheimer E, Wieland S, et al. Development of the Cochrane Collaboration's CENTRAL register of controlled clinical trials. Eval Health Prof 2002;25:38–64.

[3] Scherer RW, Langenberg P, von Elm E. Full publication of results initially presented in abstracts. The Cochrane Database Methodology Reviews 2005;2. Art. No.:MR000005 pub 2.

[4] Edwards P, Clarke M, DiGuiseppi C, et al. Identification of randomized controlled trials in systematic reviews: accuracy and reliability of screening records. Stat Med 2002;21:1635–40.

[5] Higgins JPT, Thompson SG, Deeks JJ, et al. Measuring inconsistency in meta-analyses. BMJ 2003;327:557–60.

[6] Deeks JJ, Higgins JPT, Altman DG, editors. Analysing and presenting results. In: Higgins JPT, Green S, editors. Cochrane handbook for systematic reviews of interventions 4.2.4 [updated March 2005]; Section 8. In: The Cochrane Library, Issue 2, 2005. Chichester (UK): John Wiley and Sons, Ltd; 2005.

[7] Chalmers I, Dickersin K, Chalmers TC. Getting to grips with Archie Cochrane's agenda. BMJ 1992;305:786–8.

[8] Cochrane AL. 1931–1971: a critical review, with particular reference to the medical profession. In: Medicines for the year 2000. London: Office of Health Economics; 1979. p. 1–11.

[9] Mallett S, Clarke M. How many Cochrane reviews are needed to cover existing evidence on the effects of healthcare interventions? Evid Based Med 2003;8:100–1.

[10] Chinnock P, Siegfried N, Clarke M. Is evidence-based medicine relevant to the developing world? Systematic reviews have yet to achieve their potential as a resource for practitioners in developing countries. PLoS Med 2005;2:367–9.

[11] Devereaux PJ, Bhandari M, Clarke M, et al. Need for expertise based randomised controlled trials. BMJ 2005;330:88–91.

[12] Clarke M. Doing new research? Don't forget the old: nobody should do a trial without reviewing what is known. PLoS Med 2004;1:100–2.

[13] Guenaga KF, Matos D, Castro AA, et al. Mechanical bowel preparation for elective colorectal surgery. Cochrane Database Syst Rev 2005;1:CD001544.

[14] Handoll HHG, Madhok R. Surgical interventions for treating distal radial fractures in adults. Cochrane Database Syst Rev 2003;3:CD003209.

[15] Algra A, Brilstra EH, Clarke M, et al. Endovascular coiling versus neurosurgical clipping for patients with aneurysmal subarachnoid haemorrhage. Cochrane Database Syst Rev 2005;3:CD003085.

[16] Fernandez R, Griffiths R, Ussia C. Water for wound cleansing. Cochrane Database Syst Rev 2002;4:CD003861.

SURGICAL
CLINICS OF
NORTH AMERICA

Surg Clin N Am 86 (2006) 115–128

Evaluating New Surgical Techniques in Australia: The Australian Safety and Efficacy Register of New Interventional Procedures–Surgical Experience

Guy J. Maddern, PhD, MD[a,b,*],
Philippa F. Middleton, BSc(Hons),
GradDipLibStud, MPH[a],
Rebecca Tooher, BA, PGDipAud, PhD[a],
Wendy J. Babidge, BAppSci(Hons), PhD[a,b]

[a]Australian Safety and Efficacy Register of New Interventional Procedures–Surgical
(ASERNIP–S), Royal Australasian College of Surgeons, Stepney,
South Australia, 5069 Australia
[b]Department of Surgery, University of Adelaide, The Queen Elizabeth Hospital,
Woodville Road, Woodville, SA 5011, Australia

Any process that attempts to assess and evaluate new surgical technologies needs to have significant input from the surgical community. Externally assessed and legislated processes are unlikely to enjoy much cooperation from surgeons, and have the potential for backlash from patients who feel they have been denied new, exciting technologies because of bureaucratic intervention.

Significant advantages and disadvantages are inherent in the Australian surgical system in terms of the rational introduction of new surgical techniques and technologies. The primary advantage is that all but a handful of surgeons in Australia are members of the Royal Australasian College of Surgeons. This means that any process developed and supervised by the College is likely to be widely accepted by surgeons. Furthermore, any problems that arise can be easily managed, because all surgeons in the country have ready access to the College. The main disadvantage of the Australian surgical system is that approximately 40% of all patients are privately insured,

* Corresponding author. Department of Surgery, University of Adelaide, The Queen Elizabeth Hospital, Woodville Road, Woodville, SA 5011, Australia.
  E-mail address: guy.maddern@adelaide.edu.au (G.J. Maddern).

0039-6109/06/$ - see front matter © 2006 Elsevier Inc. All rights reserved.
doi:10.1016/j.suc.2005.10.010   surgical.theclinics.com

and many surgical services are not provided under a government-supervised health service. As a result, it is more difficult for government to influence the uptake and use of new surgical procedures. Because fees paid for surgical procedures, even within the private health sector, are heavily subsidized by government, however, a lack of government support for a given technology usually means that insufficient funding is available for it to be widely taken up by the surgical community.

In 1997 the federal government of Australia, working with the Royal Australasian College of Surgeons, decided to establish the Australian Safety and Efficacy Register for New Interventional Procedures–Surgical (ASERNIP–S) to assist in the assessment of new surgical techniques and technologies. ASERNIP–S is funded from federal government sources but administered entirely by the Royal Australasian College of Surgeons. Although this arrangement required the College to provide the government with broad outcomes relating to assessment of new technologies and dissemination of this information, the day-to-day management and the crafting and drafting of reports was left entirely to the Royal Australasian College of Surgeons. ASERNIP–S commenced operations in January 1998, and has evolved substantially over time, initially focusing on the production of systematic evidence-based reviews of new surgical procedures, but gradually moving into areas such as accelerated reviews, horizon scanning, surgical audits, guideline development, and assistance in developing research protocols of new surgical technologies.

The process

The structure and processes used by ASERNIP–S have also changed over time. One of the first tasks faced by the organization was to develop a workable definition for new surgical techniques. The argument regarding what is new and what is merely surgical evolution is complex, and still remains largely unresolved. For example, it could be argued that laparoscopic cholecystectomy is not new, but is merely the same operation performed through a different series of incisions. An alternate view, which is probably more accurate, is that the change in approach substantially alters the risks and potential outcomes associated with the surgery, and thus the procedure should be considered as new.

It is perhaps less clear whether the use of a different alloy in the development of a prosthetic hip replacement or a different trochar for laparoscopic surgery constitutes a new technique or technology. Similarly, a technique that may have been suggested years ago but has only recently become more widespread as technology has improved may be viewed by the surgical community as new, even though the concept or original idea may well have been many years in gestation.

The next challenge was to form an appropriate group of individuals to oversee the process of assessing new surgical technologies. A Management

Committee was formed, with representation from the Royal Australasian College of Surgeons, consumers, Australian hospitals, Australian medical data managers, and the Cochrane Collaboration within Australia. The Management Committee plays a key role in setting the direction of ASERNIP–S assessments and in considering and ratifying reports before dissemination.

Fig. 1 illustrates the process by which systematic reviews pass through the organization. A review group of surgeons provides input into and comments on the review drafted by experienced systematic review staff at ASERNIP–S. The review is ratified by both the Management Committee and the Council of the Royal Australasian College of Surgeons. The ownership of the process by the Royal Australasian College of Surgeons and the participation of surgeons are crucial to its success. An appeals mechanism was built into this process from an early stage, because unlike other organizations attempting to look at new technologies, a broad consultation and dissemination process does not occur until after the generation of the ASERNIP–S report. This strategy was adopted to ensure that information about the safety and efficacy of new techniques could be disseminated as rapidly as possible. Disputes, though rare, have usually arisen because vested interests were present, and ASERNIP–S experience has been that a dispute may lead

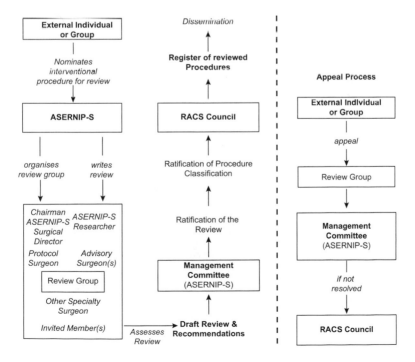

Fig. 1. The ASERNIP–S review process.

to a substantial delay, and a much slower release of information than is desirable. It seems likely that a wide consultation process before the generation of reviews could result in products with much less relevance if their dissemination is substantially delayed.

Systematic reviews

The original remit of the ASERNIP–S funding was to conduct systematic reviews of the literature relating to new interventional surgical procedures. This has been the core of activities within the organization; however, this is an expensive and time-consuming process, because finished reviews take a considerable amount of time to reach surgical consciousness and use a large volume of the resources associated with the project. Fig. 2 shows the number of systematic reviews achieved each year during the life of the ASERNIP–S program, and Table 1 documents the reviews completed to date. To hasten the uptake of new technologies and provide timely information to hospitals, patients, and surgeons, ASERNIP–S instituted a new process of "accelerated systematic review." This process enables the organization to give a more timely response to enquiries, using a more selective search regimen with probably very little loss of overall validity in the findings.

To ensure that a large volume of ASERNIP–S outputs reaches general circulation, the policy has always been to ensure that all systematic reviews were submitted to peer-reviewed journals for publication. The majority of these have been published or accepted to date (see Appendix). ASERNIP–S dissemination efforts have been supplemented by a well-designed website (http://www.surgeons.org/asernip-s), but the mainstay of surgical communication remains the body of published scientific literature. To gain maximal

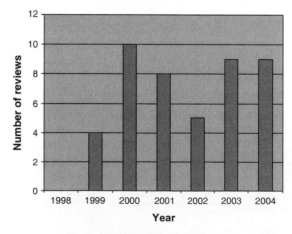

Fig. 2. Number of reviews per year.

Table 1
ASERNIP–S systematic reviews

Review name	Publication date
Minimally invasive parathyroid surgery	June 1999
Laparoscopic live-donor nephrectomy	June 1999
Lung volume reduction surgery	June 1999
Ultrasound-assisted lipoplasty	October 1999
Arthroscopic subacromial decompression using the holmium: YAG laser (reappraisal)	February 2000
Laparoscopic-assisted resection of colorectal malignancies	February 2000
Minimally invasive techniques for the relief of bladder outflow obstruction	February 2000
Percutaneous endoscopic laser discectomy (reappraisal)	February 2000
Lung volume reduction surgery (reappraisal)	May 2000
Laparoscopic adjustable gastric banding in the treatment of obesity	June 2000
Laparoscopic live-donor nephrectomy (reappraisal)	July 2000
Ultrasound-assisted lipoplasty (reappraisal)	July 2000
Minimally invasive techniques for the relief of bladder outflow obstruction (reappraisal)	November 2000
Off-pump coronary artery bypass surgery with the aid of tissue stabilizers	November 2000
Tension-free urethropexy for stress urinary incontinence: intravaginal slingplasty and the tension-free vaginal tape procedures	February 2001
Dynamic graciloplasty for the treatment of fecal incontinence	June 2001
Endoscopic modified lothrop procedure for the treatment of chronic frontal sinusitis	June 2001
Minimally invasive parathyroid surgery (reappraisal)	June 2001
Minimally invasive direct coronary artery bypass surgery—MSAC	September 2001
Off-pump coronary artery bypass surgery—MSAC	September 2001
Methods used to establish laparoscopic pneumoperitoneum	October 2001
Off-pump coronary artery bypass surgery with the aid of tissue stabilizers (reappraisal)	October 2001
Autologous fat transfer for breast augmentation	February 2002
Stapled hemorrhoidectomy	February 2002
Laparoscopic adjustable gastric banding in the treatment of obesity (reappraisal)	June 2002
Intraoperative radiotherapy in early stage breast cancer	October 2002
Radiofrequency ablation of liver tumors	October 2002
Transanal endoscopic microsurgery—MSAC	March 2003
Implantable spinal infusion devices for chronic pain and spasticity (accelerated)	May 2003
Holmium laser prostatectomy for benign prostatic hyperplasia	June 2003
Laparoscopic live donor nephrectomy (2nd reappraisal)	June 2003
Spinal cord stimulation/neurostimulation (accelerated)	June 2003
Postvasectomy testing to confirm sterility	December 2003
Surgical simulation	December 2003
Vacuum-assisted closure (accelerated)	December 2003
Intraoperative ablation for the treatment of atrial fibrillation	July 2004
Laparoscopic ventral hernia repair (accelerated)	July 2004
Technology overview: da Vinci surgical robotics system	July 2004
Adult-to-adult live-donor liver transplantation (donor outcomes)	October 2004
Adult-to-adult live-donor liver transplantation (recipient outcomes)	October 2004
Carotid percutaneous transluminal angioplasty with stenting—MSAC	Late 2004

(*continued on next page*)

Table 1 (*continued*)

Review name	Publication date
Sentinel lymph node biopsy in breast cancer (safety & efficacy)—MSAC	Late 2004
Sentinel lymph node biopsy in breast cancer (diagnostic)—MSAC	Late 2004
Unicompartmental knee arthroplasty	Late 2004

Abbreviation: MSAC, Medical Services Advisory Committee.

exposure beyond Australia, it was decided, whenever possible, to direct manuscripts to international journals unless the procedure was of particular local relevance.

The findings of systematic and accelerated reviews have largely yielded a surgical evidence base that is poor to average. Although procedures have often been found to be safe, their efficacy has not been shown to be superior the existing gold standard (where one exists), and sometimes there has been insufficient evidence to determine efficacy. Often there is a need for a substantial amount of additional research, usually in the form of randomized controlled trials, to demonstrate the new procedure's superiority or equivalence to the existing intervention. Fig. 3 summarizes the findings of the systematic reviews performed to date, and highlights the difficulty of assessing procedures early in their life cycle as opposed to when they have reached a degree of maturity, after large numbers of interventions have been performed or well-designed randomized controlled trials conducted.

Why surgery should suffer so badly from a poor evidence base has been widely discussed [1,2], but has much to do with the difficulties in obtaining true equipoise before recruiting patients into one procedure against another [3]. It is also complicated by the almost impossible task of obtaining blinding of either the patient or the surgeon, and suffers from the gradual evolution of techniques during the course of the study. Initial recruits may be subjected to an early learning curve phenomenon, and may also have a less clear grasp of the indications and complications. These difficulties will continue to plague research of new surgical procedures; however, in some instances these problems can be mitigated and alternative ways devised to try and reach valid conclusions in spite of the aforementioned difficulties [4].

In the absence of high-quality evidence from randomized controlled trials of surgical procedures, carefully collected safety and efficacy data representing the bulk of procedures conducted in Australia can provide useful information and allow assessment in their local practice context. To this end, the ASERNIP–S process has also developed a series of surgical audits. Table 2 lists the audits that have been completed or are currently being conducted within the program. In Australia, a good example of such an audit was the collection of data associated with laparoscopic renal donations from live donors for transplantation. This was a procedure hitherto unknown in Australia, despite a considerable experience in the United States. As

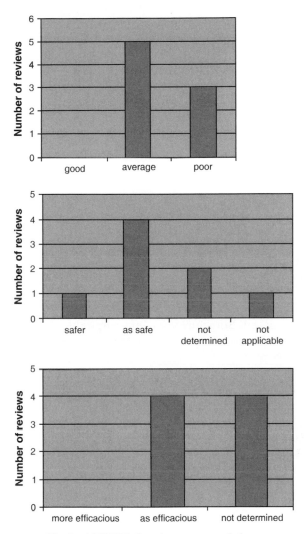

Fig. 3. ASERNIP–S review recommendations.

a result of the ASERNIP–S review, it was decided to introduce the procedure, given its intrinsic benefits in increasing the donor pool and providing less trauma to the donor, but to subject it to a surgical audit. Data were collected over a period of 4 years while centers began to take the procedure on board, and when finally summarized, it was shown that the introduction had been safe and successful within the Australian context, and the work of the audit was handed across to the Australasian Renal Transplant Registry. This work was published in the *ANZ Journal of Surgery* (see Appendix), because it was of direct interest to the Australasian surgical community. A similar audit was also conducted over an 18-month period of endoluminal

Table 2
ASERNIP–S audits

Description	Period	Type
National breast cancer audit	1998	Clinical audit
Laparoscopic live-donor nephrectomy	1998–2003	Research audit
Endoluminal repair of abdominal aortic aneurysms	1999	Research audit
Minimally invasive parathyroidectomy	1999–2000	Research audit
Deep brain stimulation	2002	Development only

vascular grafts, and a longitudinal follow-up of this cohort of patients is being conducted within the Australian vascular surgical community to determine whether the short-term benefits of endovascular aortic stents translate into a longer-term stability of the grafts being inserted.

Acceptance of the process

When establishing an enterprise such as ASERNIP–S, it is important to have an understanding of who are likely to be the potential consumers of the information produced. Surgeons, patients, hospitals, and government were identified as the groups likely to require the information generated from the ASERNIP–S process.

To date a number of surveys have been conducted of the hospitals using the ASERNIP–S process. Within Australia there are approximately 740 hospitals, all of which have been surveyed. The results of the most recent survey of these institutions (Table 3) indicated that over 60% of respondents found our notifications useful. Around one quarter had used them in the credentialing process or to change individual clinical privileges, and a further quarter had allowed or disallowed the procedure based on recommendations

Table 3
ASERNIP–S Credential Committee survey

Usefulness of ASERNIP–S Reviews	
Clinically useful/relevant/valuable	25%
Keep up to date	15%
Discuss at Medical Advisory Committee	4%
Informative or educational	18%
Not relevant to practice in our hospitals	34%
Other	4%
Resultant Decision/Action	
Allowed or disallowed a new procedure	26%
Assists implementation of new procedures	22%
Credentialing/planning process & changed application for privileges	26%
Not yet	4%
Other	13%

of a review. In general, they valued the independent nature of the assessments and used them as tools in the decision-making process.

To gauge the reaction of surgeons and their knowledge of the ASERNIP–S process, the authors also conducted a random stratified survey of 10% of College Fellows. Although there was a very low return rate, it was interesting to see that of the sample who did return responses, nearly 70% were aware of ASERNIP–S, and very few expressed negative views, although one totally shredded response was received from an obviously disenchanted surgeon! Around 85% of respondents were aware of the major roles of ASERNIP–S. The reasons given for reading our reviews were split fairly equally into personal interest, relevance to surgical specialty, or that it was a "hot topic" in surgery. The executive summary and discussion were the parts of the review read most often. The ASERNIP–S reviews were found to be user-friendly and increased the reader's understanding, but were deemed less important for decision-making. Additionally, publications of reviews in a peer-reviewed journal appeared to be a valuable method of dissemination.

Another important facet of ASERNIP–S is the provision of information to consumers. This has been in the form of summaries of all systematic reviews in an easy-to-read format that is available on the Internet. More recently a patient information sheet has been produced on several reviews for placing in the surgeons' rooms. National and specific consumer groups are also targeted with ASERNIP–S products to ensure that information is disseminated as widely as possible.

Government has also found the reports of value, and has used the ASERNIP–S information to determine the validity for government funding of a number of procedures through the Medical Services Advisory Committee (MSAC). This committee has also used ASERNIP–S to carry out audits of new procedures that had been reviewed by MSAC but for which evidence was lacking, such as transurethral needle ablation of prostates and the endoluminal aortic stent graft audit. A national clinical audit has also been facilitated at ASERNIP–S that collects information on the practice of clinicians treating early breast cancer. This is another federally-funded initiative that ultimately aims to improve breast cancer care by comparing each surgeon's practice against a set of minimum standards.

Horizon scanning

The main area of significant growth and development over recent years has been the use of horizon scanning. Horizon scanning involves detecting new techniques and technologies before their general uptake into practice. A range of methods have been used to identify these emerging surgical procedures: regular scanning of the Internet for news releases, conference presentations and journal abstracts; searching Australian and international health technology assessment sites and electronic literature databases; and regularly surveying the Fellows of the Royal Australasian College of

Surgeons (in excess of 5000 surgeons) for new and emerging technologies thought to require closer attention from ASERNIP–S. Although not all of the suggestions made by the Fellows were appropriate or relevant, many did alert the ASERNIP–S organization to technologies that required further investigation. This process has led to a large number of horizon-scanning reports being generated. Table 4 provides a list of the reports completed to date, and Fig. 4 shows the number of reports completed per year. Some of these may later become the topic of either accelerated or systematic reviews, once the procedures become more mature and suitable for such an analysis.

ASERNIP–S has recently joined the Australian and New Zealand Horizon Scanning Network to provide expertise in the area of horizon scanning in surgery while another health technology assessment agency focuses primarily on nonsurgical techniques. Both groups are working together closely, so that the format and style of the reports are similar and can be readily used by patients, hospitals, and government to advise them on future directions within the health sector.

Table 4
List of Horizon Scanning reports

Report name	Date of publication
Transaxillary thyroidectomy	September 2001
Artificial (cervical) disc replacement	October 2001
Irrigating scalpel for adhesiolysis	October 2001
Meniscal transplantation	November 2001
Electrolytic ablation of tumors	September 2002
Thyroplasty type 2	September 2002
Endoluminal stenting of the thoracic aorta	November 2002
Implantable artificial lung	November 2002
Implantable total artificial heart	December 2002
Injection snoreplasty	February 2003
Artificial intervertebral disc replacement (lumbar)	May 2003
Kyphoplasty	May 2003
Radiofrequency ablation of varicose veins	May 2003
Intradiscal electrothermal therapy	June 2003
Percutaneous endoscopic thoracic discectomy (with laser)	June 2003
Secondary transperitoneal cryotherapy for carcinoma of the prostate	June 2003
MRI guided focused ultrasound for ablation of uterine fibroids	August 2003
Essure System (Conceptus, San Carlos, California) for tubal sterilisation	February 2004
Intraoperative radiation therapy in breast cancer	April 2004
Collagen mensical implants	July 2004
Minimally invasive esophagectomy	August 2004
The Tan-Bianchi procedure and modifications	August 2004
Artificial intervertebral disc replacement (cervical)	Late 2004
Artificial intervertebral disc replacement (lumbar)	Late 2004
Endokeratoplasty	Late 2004
Stretta procedure	Late 2004

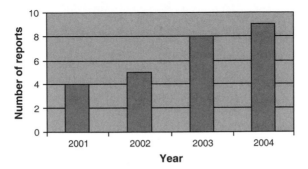

Fig. 4. Number of horizon scanning reports per year.

Future

The future for organizations such as ASERNIP–S cannot be seen in isolation. It is vital that similar enterprises are initiated in other countries around the world, and that the information gathered is readily shared among them. Given the cost and time associated with conducting systematic reviews, it is highly desirable that they be performed in a cooperative fashion, so that individual organizations do not duplicate the work of others. In this way, the overall output worldwide of high-quality systematic reviews of new interventional surgical procedures can be dramatically increased. The resources saved in collaboration would enable more of the efforts and enterprise of individual organizations to be devoted toward assessing these technologies within local environments, which are known to be different in different venues around the world. This networked, evidence-based surgical approach could also lay the groundwork for cooperative trials of interventions within different geographical locations. This arrangement might overcome some of the difficulties of conducting randomized controlled trials in surgery, including finding adequate numbers of suitable patients, and would allow other methods of data collection, such as audit, to be standardized. International cooperation in this way would also enable a better understanding of the uptake and success of procedures within different countries.

Cultural change for surgeons is not a rapid process. The ASERNIP–S experience in Australia has introduced surgeons to the trend toward surgery becoming more evidence-based. There is now general acceptance that this is a vital activity that needs to be controlled by surgeons for the benefit of their patients. The Australian experience with ASERNIP–S highlights the effectiveness of a surgeon-driven process. ASERNIP–S and Australian surgeons can act as ambassadors to the broader surgical community worldwide, educating and reinforcing the intrinsic worth of evidence-based surgical approaches being adopted by surgeons. This is far preferable to the use of government directives that may be received by surgeons as impositions, without clear relevance or consideration of the impact on clinical practice.

Appendix

ASERNIP-S peer-reviewed publications 2000

Boult M, Fraser R, Jones N, et al. Percutaneous endoscopic laser discectomy: a systematic review. Aust N Z J Surg 2000;70(7):475–9.

Reeve TS, Babidge WJ, Parkyn RF, et al. Minimally invasive surgery for primary hyperparathyroidism: a systematic review. Copublished in Arch Surg 2000;135(4):481–7, and Aust NZ J Surg 2000;70(4):244–50.

Merlin T, Scott D, Rao M, et al. The safety and efficacy of laparoscopic live donor nephrectomy: a systematic review. Transplantation 2000;70(12): 1659–66.

Wheelahan J, Scott NA, Cartmill R, et al. Minimally invasive laser techniques for prostatectomy: a systematic review. BJU Int 2000;86:805–15.

Wheelahan J, Scott NA, Cartmill R, et al. Minimally invasive non-laser thermal techniques for prostatectomy: a systematic review. BJU Int 2000;86:977–88.

EU Hernia Trialists Collaboration. Mesh compared with non-mesh methods of open groin hernia repair—systematic review of randomised controlled trials. Br J Surg 2000;87:854–9.

EU Hernia Trialists Collaboration. Laparoscopic compared with open methods of groin hernia repair—systematic review of randomised controlled trials. Br J Surg 2000;87:860–7.

EU Hernia Trialists Collaboration. Overview of randomized trials of inguinal hernia repair—a European Union concerned action. Surg Endosc 1999;13:1030–1.

Babidge W, Maddern G. Evidence-based surgery at ASERNIP-S. Can this improve quality in surgical practice? J Qual Clin Pract 2000;20:164–6.

2001

Boult M, Shimmin A, Wicks M, et al. Arthroscopic subacromial decompression with a holmium:YAG laser: review of the literature. Aust N Z J Surg 2001;71(3):172–7.

Chapman AE, Levitt MD, Hewett P, et al. Laparoscopic-assisted resection of colorectal malignancies: a systematic review. Ann Surg 2001;234(5): 590–606.

Cooter R, Chapman A, Babidge WJ, et al. Ultrasound-assisted lipoplasty: Aust N Z J Surg 2001;71(5):309–17.

Stirling GR, Babidge WJ, Peacock MJ, et al. Lung volume reduction surgery in emphysema: a systematic review. Ann Thorac Surg 2001;72(2): 641–8.

Maddern GJ. Evidence based medicine in practice–surgical. Med J Aust 2001;174(10):528–9.

Merlin T, Arnold E, Petros P, et al. A systematic review of tension-free urethropexy for stress urinary incontinence: intravaginal slingplasty and the tension-free vaginal tape procedures. BJU Int 2001;88(9): 871–80.

2002

Boult M, Babidge W, Anderson J, et al. Australian audit for the endoluminal repair of abdominal aortic aneurysm—the first 12-months. Aust N Z J Surg 2002;72(3):190–5.

Boult M, Babidge W, Roder D, et al. Issues of consent and privacy affecting the functioning of ASERNIP-S [editorial]. Aust N Z J Surg 2002; 72(8):535–6.

Boult M, Babidge W, Roder D, et al. Issues of consent and privacy affecting the functioning of ASERNIP-S. Aust N Z J Surg 2002;72(8):580–2.

Chapman A, Geerdes B, Hewett P, et al. Systematic review of dynamic graciloplasty in the treatment of faecal incontinence. Br J Surg 2002; 89(2):138–53.

Maddern GJ, Middleton PF, Grant AM. Urinary stress incontinence [editorial]. BMJ 2002;325(7368):789–90.

Scott N, Knight J, Bidstrup B, Wolfenden H, et al. Systematic review of beating heart surgery with the Octopus® Tissue Stabilizer. Eur J Cardiothorac Surg 2002;21(5):804–17.

Sutherland LM, Burchard AK, Matsuda K, et al. A systematic review of stapled haemorrhoidectomy. Arch Surg 2002;137:1395–1406.

Wagner E, Middleton P. Effects of technical editing in biomedical journals, a systematic review. JAMA 2002;287(21):2821–4.

Maddern G, Babidge W, Boult M. ASERNIP-S audits the surgical procedure endoluminal repair of abdominal aortic aneurysms. Journal of the Australasian Association for Quality in Health Care 2002;12(3):17–19.

EU Hernia Trialists Collaboration. Repair of groin hernia with synthetic mesh. Meta-analysis of randomised controlled trials. Ann Surg 2002;235(3):322–32.

2003

Campbell B, Maddern G. Safety and Efficacy of interventional procedures: scrutinising the evidence and issuing guidelines without stifling innovation. BMJ 2003;326:347–8.

Merlin T, Hiller J, Maddern G, et al. Systematic review of the safety and effectiveness of methods used to establish pneumoperitoneum in laparoscopic surgery. Br J Surg 2003;90:668–79.

Scott NA, Wormald P, Close D, et al. Endoscopic modified Lothrop procedure for the treatment of chronic frontal sinusitis: a systematic review. Otolaryngology—Head and Neck Surgery 2003;129(4):427–38.

Tooher R, Middleton P, Babidge W. Implementation of pressure ulcer guidelines: what constitutes a successful strategy? J Wound Care 2003;12(10):373–82.

2004

Chapman A, Kiroff G, Game P, et al. Laparoscopic adjustable gastric banding in the treatment of obesity: a systematic review. Surgery 2004; 135(3):326–51.

Audigé L, Reeves B, Bhandari M, et al. Methods used in orthopaedic systematic reviews. Clinical and Orthopaedic Research 2004;427:249–57.

Boult M, Babidge W, Maddern G, et al, on behalf of the Audit Reference Group. Endoluminal repair of abdominal aortic aneurysm—contemporary Australian experience. Eur J Vasc Endovasc Surg 2004;28:36–40.

Cuncins-Hearn A, Saunders C, Walsh D, et al. A systematic review of intraoperative radiotherapy in early breast cancer. Breast Cancer Res Treat 2004;85:271–80.

GRADE Working Group. Grading quality of evidence and strength of recommendations. Education and debate. BMJ 2004;328:1490–7.

Maddern GJ. Governing the ungovernable [commentary]? Aust N Z J Surg 2004;74(3):91.

Middleton PF, Sutherland L, Maddern GJ. Transanal endoscopic microsurgery: a systematic review. Dis Colon Rectum 2005;48:270–84.

Tooher R, Boult M, Maddern G, et al. Final report from the ASERNIP-S audit of laparoscopic live-donor nephrectomy. ANZ J Surg 2004; 74:961–3.

Tooher R, Griffin T, Maddern G. Vaccinations for workers in the waste handling industry. A review of the literature. Waste Manag Res 2005;23:79–86.

Tooher R, Maddern G, Simpson J. Surgical fires and alcohol-based skin preparations. Aust N Z J Surg 2004;74:382–5.

Tooher R, Middleton P, Pham C, et al. A systematic review of strategies to improve prophylaxis for venous thromboembolism in hospitals. Ann Surg 2005;241:397–415.

Tooher R, Rao M, Scott D, et al. Systematic review of laparoscopic live-donor nephrectomy. Transplantation 2004;78(3):404–14.

Tooher R, Sutherland P, Costello A. A systematic review of holmium laser prostatectomy for benign hyperplasia. J Urol 2004;17(5):1773–81.

References

[1] Audigé L, Bhandari M, Griffin D, et al. Systematic reviews of nonrandomised clinical studies in the orthopaedic literature. Clin Orthop Relat Res October 2004;(427):249–57.

[2] Green S. When should we believe the results? Quality issues in surgical research. Plenary address at the Annual Scientific Congress, Royal Australasian College of Surgeons. Melbourne, Australia, May 4, 2004.

[3] Mills N, Donovan JL, Smith M, et al. Perceptions of equipoise are crucial to trial participation: a qualitative study of men in the ProtecT study. Control Clin Trials 2003;24(3):272–82.

[4] Deeks J, Dinnes J, D'Amico R, et al. Evaluating nonrandomised intervention studies. Health Technol Assess 2003;7(27):iii–x; 1–173.

ELSEVIER
SAUNDERS

SURGICAL
CLINICS OF
NORTH AMERICA

Surg Clin N Am 86 (2006) 129–149

Evaluating Surgical Outcomes

Simon Bergman, MD, MSc[a,b],
Liane S. Feldman, MD[a,b],
Jeffrey S. Barkun, MD, MSc[a,c,*]

[a]Department of Surgery, McGill University, Royal Victoria Hospital, 687 Pine Avenue W.,
Room S10–30, Montreal, Quebec, H3A 1A1, Canada
[b]Montreal General Hospital, 1650 Cedar Avenue, Montreal, Quebec, Canada H3G 1A4
[c]Royal Victoria Hospital, 687 Pine Avenue W., Room S10-30, Montreal, Quebec,
Canada, H3A 1A1

The past decades have seen dramatic improvements in the care that is delivered to patients. Though a great many of these improvements may be traced to advances in the better understanding of disease processes, any sustained success of a new treatment approach is ultimately dependant on the impact it appears to have on patient outcome.

This article describes the process of measurement of patient outcomes, and evaluates strengths and weaknesses of several measurement tools described in the surgical literature. The authors discuss the limitations of traditional outcomes for "patient-centered" outcome assessment, although "intermediate" biological and physiological measures are not be discussed. The authors also discuss the use of "newer outcomes," in which validated measures covering various domains of patient care are used to assess the effects of surgical interventions. Finally, the authors introduce "composite outcomes" as a reflection of the multidimensional nature of modern patient care. The discussion is primarily geared toward the use of outcomes for the purposes of quality-of-care assessment and clinical research, because little information is available about the use of outcomes to guide clinical decision-making.

Outcomes as a measure of quality

Surgeons have long been pioneers in using patient outcomes to assess quality. Original efforts can be credited to Ernest A. Codman, a surgeon at the Massachusetts General Hospital in the early 1890s and a founder of the

* Corresponding author. Royal Victoria Hospital, 687 Pine Avenue W., Room S10-30, Montreal, Quebec, H3A 1A1, Canada.
E-mail address: jeffrey.barkun@muhc.mcgill.ca (J.S. Barkun).

American College of Surgeons. His peers ostracized him for his interest in using surgical outcomes to improve surgical care. He went on to found the End-Result Hospital, where he developed surgical outcomes research and became an outspoken advocate of public disclosure of complications and medical errors [1]. The use of outcomes to guide quality assessment has subsequently gained popularity throughout medicine, and this drive for assessment and accountability has been called the "third revolution in medical care" [2].

Although the widespread interest in outcomes is stimulated by a quest to improve quality of care, it is simplistic to believe that patient outcomes are synonymous with quality of care. Donabedian [3] proposed a paradigm that recognizes three components in the assessment of quality of care: structure, process, and outcome:

1. Structure includes the physical setting of the hospital or clinic, as well as the credentials of the health professionals (eg, number of nurses or respirators on a given ward or unit).
2. Process is a more complex notion that encompasses how services are provided to the patients as they move through the health care system.
3. Outcomes remain the component of Donabedian's paradigm that is best known to clinicians. In surgery, this has typically been highlighted by the presence of a normally healing wound, and the answer to that most complex of questions "how are you doing?"

A modern view of the relationship between outcomes and quality of care may best be rendered by the following statement: "outcomes are cues that prompt and motivate the assessment of process and structure in a search for causes that can be remedied" [4].

Traditional outcomes and their limitations

Surgical outcome studies have traditionally been centered on procedures rather than people who have symptoms, and on parameters that are easy to collect and that do not require special instruments or training. Outcomes data are all too often gathered, out of convenience, from a medical record or chart, and commonly in a retrospective fashion. Such data include mortality and a variety of morbidities, as well as intermediate outcomes usually related to widely available physiological and biological parameters (eg, blood tests, hemodynamic data). Such traditional outcomes can be thought of as "physician-centered," but may have several limitations in assessing outcome from the patient's perspective. For example, a comparison of percentages of complications will often be the main outcome of a published clinical report, but the patient-based significance of the data may vary tremendously (eg, patients who have an easily drained abscess after low anterior resection versus those who have ongoing, debilitating, stool incontinence). The term "Complications" can thus encompass a great variety of clinical states, and information about morbidity is often collected without standard definitions, or any attempt at a standard classification scheme. What is more, by its very nature the emphasis on recording and reporting of complications excludes the majority of patients from the outcome assessment process, because they will have failed to develop an index complication. Does this automatically signify that, in each of these cases, the operation ultimately achieved its intended goals?

Other seemingly more sophisticated traditional outcomes such as time off work, convalescence, hospital stay, physician-assessed symptom severity ("none to severe"), and physician-assessed patient satisfaction ("very dissatisfied to very satisfied"), also have limitations. They are confounded by patient comorbidity, expectations, and culture; they may lack responsiveness; and they usually rely on instruments developed ad hoc, which may not have been formally evaluated [5]. Traditional outcomes are only too often insufficient to assess the many modern procedures in which the primary aim is to improve patient well-being or quality of life [6]. Indeed, a number of physician-derived traditional outcomes are but poor surrogates of convenience for what patients and surgeons really want to know: time to full patient recovery, and the ultimate impact of a procedure on a patient's disease and life. As a consequence, recent literature has seen a justified increase in the use of patient-centered measures (functional status, physical health, emotional well-being, pain, quality of life). The purpose of these is not to replace traditional measures, but rather to add to them in order to broaden our ability to measure the impact of surgery. Although it seems intuitive that outcomes should be measured using standardized, validated, and objective instruments, the popularization of many patient centered outcomes has been hindered by a lack of familiarity with them among surgeons, and the absence of intuitive clinical interpretation. Traditional and newer patient-centered outcomes are listed in Box 1 [7].

Box 1. Traditional and patient-centered outcomes

Traditional outcomes
- Mortality
- Readmission
- Complications
- Return to work
- Other traditional measures of clinical outcomes

Patient-centered outcomes
- Functional status
- Emotional health
- Social interaction
- Cognitive function
- Degree of disability
- Other valid indicators of health

Properties of outcome measures

An outcome measure is any characteristic that would be expected to change due to an intervention. By its nature, it is a measurement, and as such, should exhibit characteristics desirable to any measurement tool: it should be objective, valid, and reliable. It should be clinically relevant for the group being studied and feasible to obtain in the population of interest. It should be able to measure changes over time in an individual or group, and exhibit qualities that facilitate statistical analysis. Furthermore, it is always best that an outcome be consistent with a biological model (Nancy E. Mayo, Montreal, Canada, personal communication, 2005). It is also important to remember that any recorded outcome may be sensitive to the influence of other variables that can affect the observed result. These are often described as confounders, and include staging of disease, patient comorbidity, expectations, and attitudes. These variables may be of such importance as to dramatically bias measured outcomes, as any clinician knows well. An ideal outcome measure should minimize the possible effect of confounding variables. Taking these variables into account is thus very important in the interpretation of reported outcomes, and this process is the subject of "risk adjustment" [8]. A formal discussion of risk adjustment is, however, outside of the scope of this article.

Outcome measures are primarily classified according to the nature of the outcome they describe (biological, physiological, or psychological) and according to their focus: generic or specific. Outcome measures can also be classified according to their mode of administration: performance or self-reported. The latter are usually questionnaires and considered subjective, whereas the former represent tasks performed by the patient and evaluated by an objective observer [9]. Performance measures have been used most often in the form of physical rehabilitation outcome measures.

Patient outcomes: using them effectively

Morbidity and mortality

Although mortality is easy to define, morbidity is not. In fact, conclusive assessments of surgical procedures remain limited by the lack of consensus on how to define and stratify complications by severity. One of the most comprehensive efforts to classify postsurgical outcomes was that of Clavien and colleagues in 1992 [10], who proposed three types of negative outcomes: complications, failure to cure (eg, residual tumor after surgery), and sequelae. In 2004, the group revised this classification to address only complications of surgery [11]. Complications are defined as "any deviation from the normal postoperative course." They are graded from I to V, according to the therapy needed to treat the complication (Table 1) [11]. This revision includes the following modifications from the original classification: the

Table 1
Classification of surgical complications

Grade	Definition
Grade I	Any deviation from the normal postoperative course without the need for pharmacological treatment or surgical, endoscopic, and radiological interventions
	Allowed therapeutic regimens are: drugs as antiemetics, antipyretics, analgetics, diuretics, electrolytes and physiotherapy. This grade also includes wound infections opened at the bedside.
Grade II	Requiring pharmacological treatment with drug other than such allowed for Grade I complications
	Blood transfusions and total parenteral nutrition are also included.
Grade III	Requiring surgical, endoscopic or radiological intervention
Grade IIIa	Intervention not under general anesthesia
Grade IIIb	Intervention under general anesthesia
Grade IV	Life-threatening complication (including CNS complications)[a] requiring IC/ICU management
Grade IVa	Single organ dysfunction (including dialysis)
Grade IVb	Multiorgan dysfunction
Grade V	Death of a patient
Suffix "d"	If the patient suffers from a complication at the time of discharge (see examples in Table 2), the suffix "d" (for "disability") is added to the respective grade of complication. This label indicates the need for a follow-up to fully evaluate the complication.

Abbreviations: CNS, central nervous system; IC, intermediate care; ICU, intensive care unit.
[a] Brain hemorrhage, ischemic stroke, subarachnoidal bleeding, but excluding transient ischemic attacks

From Dindo D, Demartines N, Clavien PA. Classification of surgical complications: a new proposal with evaluation in a cohort of 6336 patients and results of a survey. Ann Surg 2004;240(2):206; with permission.

duration of the hospital stay was no longer used as a criterion to grade complications, and life-threatening complications requiring intermediate or intensive care management were differentiated from complications treated on the ward. Complications that have the potential for long-lasting disability after the patient's discharge (eg, paralysis of a vocal cord after thyroid surgery) are highlighted by a suffix ("d" for disability). This classification was validated by its strong correlation with the duration of hospital stay, based on 6336 patients undergoing elective surgery at the University hospital of Zurich. A strong correlation was also found between the complexity of surgery (and the assumed higher complication rates) and outcome of surgery as assessed by the new classification. The acceptance and reproducibility of the classification was shown through an international survey completed by surgeons at various levels of training.

Other classifications have been proposed, including integrating the different stakeholders' perspectives; however, a classification integrating medical, payer, and patient perspectives is usually not thought to be feasible, because correlation between these different perspectives is poor [12].

Length of stay

Length of stay (LOS) is perhaps the most commonly reported measure of surgical recovery in the literature. It is easy to abstract retrospectively, and is most relevant to payers because prolonged LOS substantially increases resource use. LOS has been found to be significantly associated with both preoperative patient comorbidity and perioperative complications [13]. There are, however, many nonphysiologic variables that are involved in the decision to discharge a patient from the hospital. As a consequence, the literature reveals great discrepancies in LOS for the same procedure. In both the surgical and the nonsurgical literature, there seems to be a general trend toward shorter hospital stays in North America as compared with the rest of the world, particularly Europe. This is likely because of philosophical and economic differences at the level of health care systems. For example, in randomized studies of laparoscopic versus open appendectomy, mean LOS after open appendectomy ranges from 1 to 7 days [14]. LOS is influenced by hospital and physician culture, patient expectations, and the patient's social and economic situation. Innovative approaches to postoperative patient care such as "fast-track" surgery—with a multimodal approach to pain relief, nutrition, and early mobilization—can be shown to reduce LOS dramatically [15]. Thus, LOS should be thought of as a complex measure that reflects much more than merely the patient's actual "readiness for discharge."

Return to normal activity/return to work

Return to work and resumption of home and leisure activities are the outcomes that are usually used to define the end of the surgical recovery process (often termed "convalescence"). This information is often requested by patients in their preoperative visit to plan their postoperative care. But because there is no gold standard objective measure to define postoperative recovery for most procedures, physician guidelines about resumption of "normal" activity are based more on tradition than knowledge. Although LOS is easily determined in a retrospective fashion by chart review, return to work and return to regular activities are in fact rarely documented in routine clinical care. As such, in many surgical studies, patients are asked to report resumption of their regular activities several weeks or months following the fact, which leads to significant recall bias. This bias can be minimized with a prospective study design, and particularly with the use of diaries in which patients are asked to make note of recovery milestones as they occur. As well, "return to normal" is usually studied using nonvalidated questionnaires, produced ad hoc for the study. Authors commonly use vague terms such as "recovery of regular activities" or "return to normal" without defining how these concepts have been explained to patients in the context of postoperative recovery. In addition, patient expectations, and not only the impact of the intervention, may play a large role in the resumption of daily activities. For example, before surgery, patients randomized to a laparo-scopic inguinal hernia repair anticipated a return to full activities on average 5.5 days sooner than patients after open repair did [16]. When objective mea-sures or diaries are not used, the person assessing the outcome may also affect the result—in a study of laparoscopic versus open cholecystectomy, surgeon estimates of the "duration of convalescence" were 15% shorter than those of the nurses who objectively documented this outcome [17].

Although return to work is the outcome with the largest economic impact and is commonly used as an index of reintegration, it is prone to confound-ing and difficult to interpret. It ignores the patients who do not work or those who delay their return to work for social and other reasons, and it misclassifies those who resume work at a reduced pace or level of responsi-bility or activity. Furthermore, the time it takes to resume professional ac-tivities following surgery is influenced by many external factors, such as job satisfaction, education level, self-employment, physician's advice, and dis-ability compensation. Finally, return to work does not correlate with vali-dated measures of physical health status or functional exercise capacity [18].

Patient-centered outcome measures

Because of the above-described limitations of more conventional out-comes, greater emphasis is being placed on reporting of patient-centered outcomes. These include health-related quality of life (generic and specific), functional status, pain, and others. These outcomes are assessed using val-idated instruments to assess patient well-being in a variety of spheres. In most cases, multiple overlapping measures of outcome are used to capture different aspects of health status.

Health-related quality of life

Health-related quality of life (HRQL) is a broad construct, referring to "the physical, psychological, and social domains of health, seen as distinct areas that are influenced by a person's experiences, beliefs, expectations and perceptions" [19]. Measuring HRQL as a surgical outcome provides in-formation beyond the simple assessment of symptom severity. Two people who have the same physical health objectively may have very different qual-ity of life, owing to individual differences in expectations and adaptability [19]. In addition, although improvements in symptoms may be measurable after an intervention, the procedure may have therapeutic benefits that may not be assessed by looking strictly at symptoms. For example, after bil-iary stent placement for the palliation of malignant jaundice, ciprofloxacin is not only found to decrease the incidence of cholangitis, but also results in an improvement in the "social function" domain of patients' perceived quality of life [20].

As mentioned above, generic or specific instruments can be used to mea-sure HRQL. The advantages of generic outcomes lie in their ability to compare across different patient populations suffering from a variety of diseases. Furthermore, data allowing comparison to "normal" population values are often available for these measures (eg, SF-36, see below). The disadvantage of generic tests is that they may not be sensitive enough to detect changes in specific symptoms of diseases, unless these symptoms have an impact on overall quality of life. In addition, there may be a ceiling effect—if patients at baseline already have very good health-related quality of life, it may be hard to show an improvement related to the intervention. In contrast, specific measures are designed to look at particular disease states, or parts of the body. They may be more intuitive for patient groups or clinicians because they refer to the specific problem at hand; however, they can only be used in a narrow population and may be too narrow to measure unintended sequelae of the intervention, both good and bad [9]. A classification of HRQL instruments is given in Box 2 [21].

Generic health-related quality of life instruments. Generic measures to determine HRQL may be divided into those that use a health profile approach, and those that use a preference-based approach [21]. Different instruments vary in the format of the questions and degree of emphasis on particular domains of a person's health.

Health profile-based instruments provide scores within various domains of health (ie, physical, psychological, and social functioning) so that the impact of a particular intervention on HRQL can be specifically defined. Several also provide summary scores. Table 2 [22–28] summarizes several generic health profile-based measures that have been used in digestive surgery. Their content varies considerably, as do the time required for administration and the way in which they are analyzed. Most rely on a weighted scoring scheme, which is calculated with the use of a computer program. In general, these profiles were developed and tested in patients who had chronic conditions, and their reliability and validity for measuring acute changes in the perioperative period may not be proven. For example, the

---

Box 2. Health-related quality of life instruments

Generic *instruments*
- Health profiles
- Preference-based measures

Specific *instruments*
- Disease-specific (eg, diabetes)
- Population-specific (eg, frail elderly)
- Function-specific (eg, sexual function)
- Condition or problem-specific (eg, pain)

usefulness of the Nottingham Health Profile (NHP) to assess health in the general population and in patients who have more minor problems is limited by a "floor effect." Indeed, many people score 0 or "no problems," and it is then difficult to observe a potential improvement [21]. In general, however, these instruments have been extensively tested for reliability, validity, and sensitivity to change in a variety of patient populations [29].

The SF-36 is by far the most frequently used generic health profile measure, and it will thus be described in more detail. The SF-36 questionnaire has been widely validated and uses a 36-item, health-related quality of life questionnaire. Answers to specific items allow the computation of scores in eight distinct health domains:

1. Physical functioning (PF) assesses limitations to daily activities.
2. Role–physical (RP) identifies limitations in work or activities caused by physical health,
3. Bodily pain (BP) grades pain and limitations therefrom.
4. General health (GH) examines health perception.
5. Vitality (VT) comprises fatigue and energy scales.
6. Social functioning (SF) assesses social limitations.
7. Role–emotional (RE) identifies limitation in work or activities due to emotional health.
8. Mental health (MH), grades feelings of anxiety and depression.

These eight scores range from 0 to 100, with a higher score indicating better health. A difference of 5 points in a particular domain is considered a minimal clinically and socially relevant change, whereas a 10-point difference is moderate. Two summary composite scores, the physical component summary (PCS) and the mental component summary (MCS) are calculated from contributions of varying weights by the eight domains: PF, RP, BP, and GH are the main contributors to PCS, whereas RE, MH, VT, and SF are the main contributors to the MCS. Both summary scores are standardized to have a mean of 50 and a standard deviation of 10. The SF-36 was introduced in 1988 and has since been translated for use in over 50 countries; it has been used to evaluate health-related quality of life in over 130 diseases and conditions covering well over 1000 publications. A review of SF-36 validation studies is beyond the scope of this article, but the SF-36 user's manuals are excellent references that describe in detail the reliability and validity of this instrument [30,31].

The SF-36 has been shown to have very good internal consistency, and to correlate well with other quality of life instruments such as the NHP, the EuroQol (see below), and disease-specific instruments. It is sensitive to change following several different types of medical interventions [9]. Although most of the validation work was done in chronic disease states, there are many surgical studies that have demonstrated its discriminating responsiveness to change. For example, quality of life was improved from baseline at 3 months following either laparoscopic or open hernia repair with

Table 2
Generic HRQL measures that have been used as surgical outcomes

HRQL measures	Short-Form 36 (SF-36)	Nottingham Health Profile (NHP)	Sickness Impact Profile (SIP)	Quality of life index (QLI)	Quality of Well Being Scale (QWBS)	EuroQol (EQ-5D)
Where to find the instrument	www.sf-36.org [22]	McDowell et al [23]	www.outcomes-trust.org/ instruments. htm#SIP [24]	www.uic.edu/orgs/ qli/index.htm [25]	www.outcomes-trust.org/ instruments. htm#QWB [26]	www.euroqol.org [27]
Purpose	Designed as indicator of perceived health status for use in general population	Measures perceived health status in general population	Measure of how illness changes daily activities and behaviors	Measures quality of life in terms of satisfaction with life	Measures well-being based on standardized preferences associated with level of functioning	Provides a health profile and an index value of health status
Description Domains	Health profile Physical functioning Role limitations due to physical problems Bodily pain General health perceptions Vitality Social functioning Role limitations due to emotional problems Mental health Health transition	Health profile Energy level Emotional reactions Physical mobility Pain Social isolation Sleep	Health profile Ambulation Mobility Body care and movement Communication Alertness behavior Emotional behavior Social interaction Sleep and rest Eating Work Home management Recreation and pastimes	Health profile Health and functioning Psychological/ spiritual Social and economic Family	Preference-based Mobility Physical activity Social activity Symptoms/problems	Preference-based Mobility Self-care Usual activity Pain/discomfort Anxiety/depression
Summary scales	Physical and mental component summary scales		Physical and psychosocial dimensions	Total quality of life score	Single index value	Single index value and visual analog scale (VAS)

Scoring	Weighted; eight domain scores (0–100) and overall physical and mental health component summary scores	Weighted; six section scores from 0 (no problems) to 100 (all items checked)	Weighted; 12 categories and two dimensions scored from 0 (no dysfunction) to 100 (maximal dysfunction)	Weighted; total quality of life score and four subscales. Scores for each range from 0–30	Weighted scores with transformation according to a formula from 0 (death) to 1 (optimal health)	Conversion of health state to utility value from 0 to 1
Administration	Self, interviewer	Self, interviewer	Self, interviewer	Self, interviewer	Interviewer	Self, interviewer
Time to complete	7–10 minutes	5–10 minutes	20–30 minutes	10 minutes	10–30 minutes	2–3 minutes
Number of items	36	38	136	66	4	5 plus VAS
Alternative forms	SF-36: 4 week recall, 1 week recall; 12 item SF-12 and 8-item SF-8		Shorter forms developed for some illnesses	Different versions for various conditions	Self-administered QWB-SA scale	

Data from **Refs. [6,9,21,28].**

mesh [32]. A randomized controlled study of laparoscopic versus open gastric bypass showed that 1 month following surgery, the physical functioning, social functioning, general health, and bodily pain were significantly greater in the laparoscopic group. At 3 months, the laparoscopic group had reached United States population norms, but physical functioning in the open group was still well below these norms [33]. The SF-36 can also detect change secondary to complications. Boerma and colleagues [34] demonstrated persistence of quality of life impairment 5 years following iatrogenic bile duct injury from laparoscopic cholecystectomy. In patients having undergone colectomy for benign disease, the presence of incisional hernia or small bowel obstruction was predictive of lower scores in several of the physical subdomains as well as in the mental component summary score [35].

Preference-based measures appear less frequently than health profiles in the surgical literature, but three preference-based measures that have been used are the Quality of Well Being Scale (QWBS), the EuroQol Instrument (EQ-5D), and the Health Utilities Index-3 (HUI-3). The EuroQoL has two sections: the EQ-5D index and the EQ-5D visual analog scale (VAS). The EQ-5D index comprises five dimensions; each assessed using a three-point scale reflecting "no problem," "some problem," and "extreme problem." The EQ-5D can thus identify a total of 243 possible health states. In contrast, the HUI-3, developed at McMasters University, describes 972,000 unique health states. In both cases, each possible combination of responses describes a unique health state, which is converted, using a formula, to a utility value ranging from 0 to 1.0. For the EQ-5D, the formula for the population-weighted health index was obtained from the general population using the time-tradeoff technique, in which subjects are asked how much time in a state of perfect health they consider equivalent to time in various health states (for example, a subject might consider 10 years of perfect health to be equivalent to 12 years with severe back pain). The EQ-5D also gives a self-rated global assessment of health status based on a 20-cm visual analog scale (VAS), ranging from 0 (best health state) to 100 (worst possible health state). The EQ-5D was concurrently developed in five languages (Dutch, UK English, Finnish, Norwegian, and Swedish). It has the major advantage of having been designed to be self-administered, is short enough to be used in conjunction with other measures, and has been validated in a great many languages and cultures.

Overall, preference-based measures are particularly useful in cost effectiveness studies, in which the cost of an intervention is compared with its outcome and expressed in quality-adjusted life-years (QALYs, see below).

Disease-specific health-related quality of life instruments. For specific conditions, a general health survey may not be sensitive enough to capture changes related to a surgical intervention. Disease-specific questionnaires may be more responsive, and may encompass more specifically symptoms addressed by the intervention. In addition, information about how the intervention affects specific aspects of the condition may be obtained. These surveys include questions assessing the severity of specific symptoms, and also the impact of those symptoms on the individual's quality of life. In so doing, they go beyond simple "Likert scales": categorical scales assessing symptom severity (eg, "How bad is your heartburn: none/mild/moderate/ severe?"). Likert scales are limited in their range of responses, do not allow for a composite assessment of the often multiple symptoms associated with various conditions, and do not assess the impact of the symptom on the patient's quality of life. Overall scores are produced by the questionnaires, but the impact of the intervention on any specific symptom addressed in the questionnaire can also be individually analyzed in a descriptive fashion. A systematic review of HRQL assessment in minimally invasive surgery, with evidenced-based guidelines of which instruments to use for a variety of procedures, has been published by the European Association for Endoscopic Surgery [29]. Examples of some quality of life instruments relevant to digestive surgery are listed in Box 3.

Functional outcomes: activities, disability, and measuring recovery

Every surgical procedure involves a period of recovery. In the immediate postoperative period, fatigue, pain, and other factors impact on patients' abilities to fully resume their usual roles and activities, including those related to work, family and leisure; however, few studies in the surgical literature use validated measures of function, activities, and quality of life to measure this period of disability. They rely instead on length of stay, or patient-reported "return to normal" or "return to work" to define recovery. As discussed above, although these outcomes are relatively easy to collect, they are influenced by many factors outside of the investigator's control. These factors include the type of work or leisure activities, the culture of the health care system, patient and surgeon expectations, and the patient's social situation and the presence of comorbid conditions. Because a baseline level of activity is often not measured, changes during the recovery period cannot be compared objectively. Ideally, in assessing the period of postoperative disability, a measure would be used at baseline, and repeated at intervals during the postoperative period. The time required for the measure to return to the baseline level would then be the time required for recovery ("convalescence").

Disability can be assessed using self-reported (questionnaires) or performance-based methods.

Questionnaires assessing disability include those evaluating the ability to perform "activities of daily living," such as bathing, dressing, and moving around the house, and "instrumental activities of daily living," such as preparing meals and managing finances. These activities have been shown to decrease in elderly patients after major abdominal surgery, requiring 3 to 6 months to return to baseline levels [52]. These measures, though, are suited primarily for elderly or institutionalized patients. Assessment of physical

---

Box 3. Quality of life instruments for digestive surgery

Foregut
- Gastrointestinal Quality of Life Index (GIQLI) [36]
- Gastrointestinal Symptom Rating Scale (GSRS) [37]
- Quality of life in Reflux and Dyspepsia Patients (QOLRAD) [38]
- Gastroesophageal Reflux Disease-Health Related Quality of Life (GERD-HRQL) [39]
- European Organization for Research and Treatment of Cancer Stomach Module (EORTC-QLQ-STO22) [40]

Colorectal
- Functional Assessment of Cancer Therapy-Colorectal (FACT-C) [41]
- Fecal Incontinence Quality of Life Scale (FIQL) [42]
- European Organization for Research and Treatment of Cancer (EORTC QLQ-C30) [43]
- European Organization for Research and Treatment of Cancer-Colorectal Cancer (EORTC QLQ-CR38) [44]
- Inflammatory Bowel Disease Questionnaire (IBDQ) [45]
- Crohn's Disease Activity Index (CDAI) [46]

Hepatobiliary and pancreatic
- European Organization for Research and Treatment of Cancer (EORTC QLQ-C30) [43]
- European Organization for Research and Treatment of Cancer-Liver Metastases from Colorectal Cancer module (EORTC QLQ-LMC21) [47]
- Gastrointestinal Quality of life Index (GIQLI) [36]
- Functional Assessment of Cancer Therapy-Hepatobiliary (FACT-Hep) [48]
- Chronic Liver Disease Questionnaire (CLDQ) [49]

Obesity
- Impact of Weight on Quality of Life-Lite Questionnaire (IWQOL-lite) [50]
- Bariatric Analysis and Reporting System (BAROS) [51]
- Gastrointestinal Quality of Life Index (GIQLI) [36]

---

activity for older adults living in the community can be done using surveys such as the Community Healthy Activities Model Program for Seniors (CHAMPS) [53], which assesses time spent on performance on a list of physical activities over a 1-week period, which can then be converted into metabolic equivalents. It has yet to be validated as a measure of recovery after abdominal surgery, however. The absence of an accepted self-reported measure of postoperative disability prompted McCarthy and colleagues [5] to create a new instrument, the Activities Assessment Scale (AAS). This was developed and used in a large randomized trial of laparoscopic versus open inguinal hernia repair, and was shown to be reliable, valid, and responsive in that patient population.

Performance-based measures of disability require an assessor to measure function of a specific task and set of tasks. Lawrence and coworkers [52] used "hand grip strength, "timed up and go" (the time required to rise from a chair, walk 3 meters, and return to the chair), and "functional reach test" (an assessment of postural control) to assess functional recovery after major abdominal surgery in the elderly. The timed up and go test returned to baseline at 6 weeks; the functional reach by 3 months, and the hand grip test had not yet returned to normal by 6 months after abdominal surgery [52]. Timed walking tests, developed originally as simple measures to assess exercise tolerance in patients who have pulmonary disease, have also been used as measures of functional exercise capacity in the perioperative period. In the 6-minute walk test (6MWT), for example, the distance walked in a 6-minute period is recorded [54]. This evaluates the ability to maintain the moderate level of walking required to perform activities of daily living. The 6MWT, which can be performed in the in-patient setting, has been found to be sensitive to change after colorectal surgery, with only 50% of patients back to baseline after 6 weeks [55], and after laparoscopic donor nephrectomy, where only 37% had returned to baseline after 4 weeks [18]. The 2-minute walk test (2MWT) is a quicker alternative to the 6MWT, and it is also sensitive to change following surgery. Physical motor activity can be measured continuously using a small monitor worn on the wrist or ankle. It senses motion via an internal accelerometer and continuously records the information, which is then downloaded onto a personal computer for analysis. Activity level, caloric expenditure, duration of activity, and sleep patterns can also be monitored. Data analysis, however, can be cumbersome, and extensive validation of this approach, as well as its relevance to other measures of recovery, is not yet available.

Pain

Most pain assessment tools are unidimensional generic psychological measures, which consider pain intensity only by asking "how much pain do you have?" There are several ways to record an answer; the three most widely used scales are: visual analog scales (VAS), numerical rating scales (NRS), and verbal rating scales (VRS). Most VAS consist of a 10-centimeter (100 mm) line drawn between two anchors, "no pain" and "worst possible pain," on which patients mark an "X" to indicate their level of pain. There is no gold standard for pain measurement, but VAS are very frequently used in the surgical literature to compare different postoperative pain management strategies. The minimum clinically important difference ranges between 10 and 30 mm on the scale mentioned above, depending on whether the difference in pain occurs at the lower or higher end of the scale, which is a significant limitation for this type of instrument. Furthermore, several iterations may be needed for optimal assessment of pain. Finally, VAS may not be very practical in certain patient populations, such as the elderly and the less literate, because of potential motor or cognitive limitations.

Simpler and more intuitive alternatives are the NRS and VRS types, which are preferred over VAS by most patients and physicians, and are comparable to VAS in their sensitivity and reliability. One NRS requires patients to select an integer between 0 and 10 (anchored by similar extremes of pain as VAS) that best corresponds to their level of pain. Reported minimum clinically important differences for NRS are similar to those of VAS. One VRS grades current pain on an ordinal scale (eg, 0 = no pain, 1 = some pain, 2 = considerable pain, 3 = pain that could not be more severe). Although the range of response is equivalent to that of VAS, data are discrete as opposed to continuous, and these scales do not possess ratio scale characteristics. This limits analysis of the results such that pre- and postintervention scores cannot be subtracted or divided, but only interpreted as more or less painful.

Multidimensional pain questionnaires offer greater insight into the different qualities of the pain experience than do single-item measures, which only focus on intensity. The drawback is that they take longer to administer and are more complex to score. In the original McGill Pain Questionnaire (MPQ), patients describe their subjective pain by selecting one word from a series of adjectives in 20 word sets among three categories (sensory, affective, and evaluative). The value for each word chosen is based on its position in the word set. Pain intensity is also rated using a VRS [56]. The short-form MPQ consists of a list of 15 descriptors rated on an intensity scale (0 = none to 3 = severe) [57]. The MPQ has been shown to be valid and reliable in a multitude of acute pain studies and in a great many languages. Other multidimensional tools include the Descriptor Differential Scale, in which verbal descriptors are rated on a 21-point scale (from negative to positive) [58], and the Westhaven-Yale Multidimensional Pain Inventory, used mostly in chronic pain, which broadly addresses the effect of pain on general functioning [59].

Patient satisfaction

Patient satisfaction is an outcome that has received only peripheral attention in the past, but is now starting to gain importance. By contrasting their expectations and preferences with the interpretation of the care they have received, individuals are essentially able to rate the experience of treatment of disease along the three Donabedian axes of quality of care (see above). If used appropriately, patient satisfaction questionnaires could represent a powerful tool by allowing patient empowerment, by offering physicians immediate patient-centered feedback, and by shaping policy at an administrative level. In the surgical literature, most satisfaction assessments are limited to one or two questions (eg, "How satisfied were you with your operation?") and less commonly involve multiple questions, which have been shown to be more reliable and sensitive to treatment differences than single-item measures. This may occur because these surveys may yield widely variable scores depending on how questions are formulated, which may be minimized by multi-item questionnaires. Domains most often assessed include overall satisfaction, outcomes of treatment, disease-related information, treatment-related discomfort, product design or appearance, and convenience [60]. To measure these outcomes, ordinal scales are often used, and range from "not at all satisfied" to "very satisfied."

Unfortunately, patient satisfaction questionnaires are still in their infancy, and mostly are either poorly validated or unvalidated tools. Their development often relies only on what investigators believe to be the factors with the most impact on patient satisfaction. The tools that have been rigorously validated are often too disease- or treatment-specific to apply to other conditions. An example is the Quality of Recovery Score, which measures satisfaction of recovery from anesthesia [61]. That they are not psychometrically sound tools may explain why most reported satisfaction ratings are usually high and thus poorly discriminatory. Although patient satisfaction questionnaires should be a part of patient-centered outcome assessment, many questions remain regarding their methodology and significance, and they should be interpreted cautiously.

Composite measures

The use of composite measures to express outcomes has increased significantly over the past years, especially in the cardiovascular literature. A quick search of medical terms for "composite outcomes" through online abstracts yielded an increase from 12 citations to 94 over the past 8 years. Composite outcomes are usually based on a summation of traditional outcomes (eg, in cardiac surgery: deaths, plus myocardial infarctions, plus heart failure, plus elevation of serum troponin levels) [62], but may be far more complex. In fact, a broader definition of composite outcomes might even include QALYs: these are the mathematical product of duration of life and a utility score reflecting the life expectancy gained, adjusted for altered quality of life. Composite outcomes are most often used in randomized trials, and in two contexts: if a single dominating outcome cannot be clearly defined, or to obtain a positive statistical result with a smaller sample size. Although they are supported by some authors, many have debated their use because they are rarely validated [62]. Nevertheless, the more clearly a composite outcome is associated with a primary objective or disease process, the less the problem with their interpretation. Although a complete discussion of composite outcomes is beyond the scope of this article, the authors refer to a particular technique that has been coined "clinical benefit" [63]. Traditionally, physicians have reported patient outcomes as a collection of means or percentages of single distinct end points (eg, death, size of tumor, wound infection rates, and so forth) This has often been a decision of convenience that does not reflect the multidimensional aspect of individual patient care. In actual fact, clinicians are more often interested in combinations of outcomes, which reflect the way in which disparate information is used to make clinical decisions. For example, following groin hernia repair, chronic groin pain and recurrent hernia are arguably two of the most significant outcomes. They may be totally independent. In assessing which of two techniques of hernia repair is superior, study results would traditionally compare percentages of hernia recurrence and percentages of patients who had pain, as associated with each repair. But how many patients actually develop either one or both of these outcomes? An alternative way of detecting superiority of the type of repair would be to consider four patient groups, reflecting the way in which clinicians might approach the problem. A given patient may have developed either both complications, or only one of the complications, and in fact may have developed neither of these complications. One could then argue that a truly successful result should be applied to this latter group alone ("winners"). The superior surgical technique should therefore in fact be the one associated with the greatest percentage of winners. This example illustrates the need to think of patient outcomes in terms of clinical syndromes rather than isolated symptoms, which mimics daily clinical care more closely than a conventional approach. This is an example of the construct behind the concept of clinical benefit. This technique has been used in oncology and in solid organ transplantation, but it still requires widespread validation [64,65].

Summary

The authors have attempted to describe some the shortcomings of existing outcomes in surgery and to introduce more patient-based end points. Strategies to evaluate outcomes in a fashion that more closely mimics clinical decision-making may hold a promise to improve our ability to draw conclusions from published trials.

References

[1] Neuhauser D. Ernest Amory Codman MD. Qual Saf Health Care 2002;11(1):104–5.
[2] Relman AS. Assessment and accountability: the third revolution in medical care. N Engl J Med 1988;319(18):1220–2.
[3] Donabedian A. Evaluating the quality of medical care. Milbank Mem Fund Q 1966; 44(3 Suppl):166–206.
[4] Hammermeister KE, Johnson R, Marshall G, et al. Continuous assessment and improvement in quality of care. A model from the Department of Veterans Affairs cardiac surgery. Ann Surg 1994;219(3):281–90.

[5] McCarthy M, Jonasson O, Chang C, et al. Assessment of patient functional status after surgery. J Am Coll Surg 2005;201:171–8.

[6] Liu JY, Birkmeyer JD. Measuring surgical outcomes. In: Souba WW, Wilmore DW, editors. Surgical research. San Diego (CA): Academic Press; 2001. p. 101–13.

[7] Lorenz W, Troidl H, Solomkin JS, et al. Second step: testing-outcome measurements. World J Surg 1999;23(8):768–80.

[8] Pillai SB, van Rij AM, Williams S, et al. Complexity- and risk-adjusted model for measuring surgical outcome. Br J Surg 1999;86(12):1567–72.

[9] Finch E, Brooks D, Stratford PW, et al. Physical rehabilitation outcome measures: a guide to enchanced clinical decision making. 2nd edition. Hamilton (Canada): BC Decker; 2002.

[10] Clavien PA, Sanabria JR, Strasberg SM. Proposed classification of complications of surgery with examples of utility in cholecystectomy. Surgery 1992;111(5):518–26.

[11] Dindo D, Demartines N, Clavien PA. Classification of surgical complications: a new proposal with evaluation in a cohort of 6336 patients and results of a survey. Ann Surg 2004; 240(2):205–13.

[12] Hunt CM, Camargo CA Jr, Dominitz JA, et al. Effect of postoperative complications on health and employment following liver transplantation. Clin Transplant 1998;12(2):99–103.

[13] Collins TC, Daley J, Henderson WH, et al. Risk factors for prolonged length of stay after major elective surgery. Ann Surg 1999;230(2):251–9.

[14] Sauerland S, Lefering R, Neugebauer EA. Laparoscopic versus open surgery for suspected appendicitis [update of Cochrane Database Syst Rev 2002;(1):CD001546; pmid: 11869603]. Cochrane Database Syst Rev 2004;(4):CD001546.

[15] Basse L, Hjort Jakobsen D, Billesbolle P, et al. A clinical pathway to accelerate recovery after colonic resection. Ann Surg 2000;232(1):51–7.

[16] Barkun JS, Wexler MJ, Hinchey EJ, et al. Laparoscopic versus open inguinal herniorrhaphy: preliminary results of a randomized controlled trial. Surgery 1995;118(4):703–9 [discussion: 9–10].

[17] Barkun JS, Barkun AN, Sampalis JS, et al. Randomised controlled trial of laparoscopic versus mini cholecystectomy. The McGill gallstone treatment group. Lancet 1992;340(8828): 1116–9.

[18] Bergman S, Feldman LS, Mayo NE, et al. Measuring surgical recovery: The study of laparoscopic live donor nephrectomy. American Journal of Transplantation 2005;5:2489–95.

[19] Testa MA, Simonson DC. Assesment of quality-of-life outcomes. N Engl J Med 1996; 334(13):835–40.

[20] Chan G, Barkun J, Barkun AN. The role of ciprofloxacin in prolonging polyethylene biliary stent patency: a multicenter double blinded effectiveness study. J Gastrointest Surg 2005;9:481–8.

[21] Coons SJ, Rao S, Keininger DL, et al. A comparative review of generic quality-of-life instruments. Pharmacoeconomics 2000;17(1):13–35.

[22] Short-form 36. Available at: www.sf-36.org. Accessed September 1, 2005.

[23] McDowell I, Newell C. Measuring health: a guide to rating scales and questionnaires. 2nd edition. New York: Oxford University Press; 1996.

[24] Sickness impact profile. Available at: http://www.outcomes-trust.org/instruments.htm#SIP. Accessed September 1, 2005.

[25] Quality of life index. Available at: www.uic.edu/orgs/qli/index.htm. Accessed September 1, 2005.

[26] Quality of well-being scale. Available at: http://www.outcomes-trust.org/instruments.htm# QWB. Accessed September 1, 2005.

[27] EuroQol EQ-5D. Available at: www.euroqol.org. Accessed September 1, 2005.

[28] American Thoracic Society. Quality of life and functional status instruments. Available at: www.atsqol.org/qinst.asp. Accessed September 1, 2005.

[29] Korolija D, Sauerland S, Wood-Dauphinee S, et al. Evaluation of quality of life after laparoscopic surgery: evidence-based guidelines of the European Association for Endoscopic Surgery. Surg Endosc 2004;18(6):879–97.

[30] Ware JE, Kosinski M, Gandek B. Sf-36 health survey: manual and interpretation guide. Lincoln (RI): QualityMetric Incorporated; 2003.

[31] Ware JE Jr, Kosinski MA. Sf-36 physical and mental health summary scales: a manual for users of version 1. 2nd edition. Lincoln (RI): QualityMetric Incorporated; 2004.

[32] Neumayer L, Giobbie-Hurder A, Jonasson O, et al. Open mesh versus laparoscopic mesh repair of inguinal hernia. N Engl J Med 2004;350(18):1819–27.

[33] Nguyen NT, Goldman C, Rosenquist CJ, et al. Laparoscopic versus open gastric bypass: a randomized study of outcomes, quality of life, and costs. Ann Surg 2001;234(3):279–89.

[34] Boerma D, Rauws EA, Keulemans YC, et al. Impaired quality of life 5 years after bile duct injury during laparoscopic cholecystectomy: a prospective analysis. Ann Surg 2001;234(6): 750–7.

[35] Thaler K, Dinnewitzer A, Mascha E, et al. Long-term outcome and health-related quality of life after laparoscopic and open colectomy for benign disease. Surg Endosc 2003;17(9): 1404–8.

[36] Eypasch E, Williams JI, Wood-Dauphinee S, et al. Gastrointestinal Quality of Life Index: development, validation and application of a new instrument. Br J Surg 1995;82(2):216–22.

[37] Svedlund J, Sjodin I, Dotevall G. GSRS—a clinical rating scale for gastrointestinal symptoms in patients with irritable bowel syndrome and peptic ulcer disease. Dig Dis Sci 1988; 33(2):129–34.

[38] Wiklund IK, Junghard O, Grace E, et al. Quality of life in reflux and dyspepsia patients. Psychometric documentation of a new disease-specific questionnaire (QOLRAD). Eur J Surg Suppl 1998;(583):41–9.

[39] Velanovich V, Vallance SR, Gusz JR, et al. Quality of life scale for gastroesophageal reflux disease. J Am Coll Surg 1996;183(3):217–24.

[40] Vickery CW, Blazeby JM, Conroy T, et al. Development of an EORTC disease-specific quality of life module for use in patients with gastric cancer. Eur J Cancer 2001;37(8): 966–71.

[41] Ward WL, Hahn EA, Mo F, et al. Reliability and validity of the functional assessment of cancer therapy-colorectal (FACT-C) quality of life instrument. Qual Life Res 1999;8(3): 181–95.

[42] Rockwood TH, Church JM, Fleshman JW, et al. Fecal Incontinence Quality of Life scale: quality of life instrument for patients with fecal incontinence. Dis Colon Rectum 2000; 43(1):9–16.

[43] Aaronson NK, Ahmedzai S, Bergman B, et al. The European Organization for Research and Treatment of Cancer QLQ-C30: a quality-of-life instrument for use in international clinical trials in oncology. J Natl Cancer Inst 1993;85(5):365–76.

[44] Sprangers MA, te Velde A, Aaronson NK. The construction and testing of the EORTC colorectal cancer-specific quality of life questionnaire module (QLQ-CR38). European Organization for Research and Treatment of Cancer Study Group on Quality of Life. Eur J Cancer 1999;35(2):238–47.

[45] Guyatt G, Mitchell A, Irvine EJ, et al. A new measure of health status for clinical trials in inflammatory bowel disease. Gastroenterology 1989;96(3):804–10.

[46] Best WR, Becktel JM, Singleton JW, et al. Development of a Crohn's disease activity index. National Cooperative Crohn's Disease Study. Gastroenterology 1976;70(3):439–44.

[47] Kavadas V, Blazeby JM, Conroy T, et al. Development of an EORTC disease-specific quality of life questionnaire for use in patients with liver metastases from colorectal cancer. Eur J Cancer 2003;39(9):1259–63.

[48] Heffernan N, Cella D, Webster K, et al. Measuring health-related quality of life in patients with hepatobiliary cancers: The Functional Assessment of Cancer Therapy-Hepatobiliary questionnaire. J Clin Oncol 2002;20(9):2229–39.

[49] Younossi ZM, Guyatt G, Kiwi M, et al. Development of a disease specific questionnaire to measure health related quality of life in patients with chronic liver disease. Gut 1999;45(2): 295–300.

[50] Kolotkin RL, Crosby RD. Psychometric evaluation of the impact of weight on quality of life-lite questionnaire (IWQOL-lite) in a community sample. Qual Life Res 2002;11(2): 157–71.

[51] Oria HE, Moorehead MK. Bariatric analysis and reporting outcome system (BAROS). Obes Surg 1998;8(5):487–99.

[52] Lawrence VA, Hazuda HP, Cornell JE, et al. Functional independence after major abdominal surgery in the elderly. J Am Coll Surg 2004;199(5):762–72.

[53] Stewart AL, Mills KM, King AC, et al. CHAMPS physical activity questionnaire for older adults: outcomes for interventions. Med Sci Sports Exerc 2001;33(7):1126–41.

[54] Laboratories ATSCoPSfCPF. ATS statement: guidelines for the six-minute walk test. Am J Respir Crit Care Med 2002;166(1):111–7.

[55] Carli F, Mayo N, Klubien K, et al. Epidural analgesia enhances functional exercise capacity and health-related quality of life after colonic surgery: results of a randomized trial. Anesthesiology 2002;97(3):540–9.

[56] Melzack R. The McGill Pain Questionnaire: major properties and scoring methods. Pain 1975;1(3):277–99.

[57] Melzack R. The short-form McGill Pain Questionnaire. Pain 1987;30(2):191–7.

[58] Gracely RH, Kwilosz DM. The Descriptor Differential Scale: applying psychophysical principles to clinical pain assessment. Pain 1988;35(3):279–88.

[59] Kerns RD, Turk DC, Rudy TE. The West Haven-Yale Multidimensional Pain Inventory (WHYMPI). Pain 1985;23(4):345–56.

[60] Weaver M, Patrick DL, Markson LE, et al. Issues in the measurement of satisfaction with treatment. Am J Manag Care 1997;3(4):579–94.

[61] Myles PS, Hunt JO, Nightingale CE, et al. Development and psychometric testing of a quality of recovery score after general anesthesia and surgery in adults. Anesth Analg 1999;88(1): 83–90.

[62] Freemantle N, Calvert M, Wood J, et al. Composite outcomes in randomized trials: greater precision but with greater uncertainty? JAMA 2003;289(19):2554–9.

[63] Ballatori E, Del Favero A, Roila F. Clinical benefit as a primary efficacy endpoint. J Clin Oncol 1998;16(2):803–4.

[64] Cantarovich M, Elstein E, de Varennes B, et al. Clinical benefit of neoral dose monitoring with cyclosporine 2-hr post-dose levels compared with trough levels in stable heart transplant patients. Transplantation 1999;68(12):1839–42.

[65] Burris HA 3rd, Moore MJ, Andersen J, et al. Improvements in survival and clinical benefit with gemcitabine as first-line therapy for patients with advanced pancreas cancer: a randomized trial. J Clin Oncol 1997;15(6):2403–13.

ELSEVIER
SAUNDERS

SURGICAL
CLINICS OF
NORTH AMERICA

Surg Clin N Am 86 (2006) 151–168

Ethical Issues in Evidence-Based Surgery

Ingrid Burger, BS[a],
Jeremy Sugarman, MD, MPH, MA[a,b,c],
Steven N. Goodman, MD, PhD[b,d,e,*]

[a]*Department of Health Policy and Management,
Johns Hopkins Bloomberg School of Public Health, Baltimore, MD 21205, USA*
[b]*Phoebe Berman Bioethics Institute, The Johns Hopkins University,
Baltimore, MD 21205, USA*
[c]*Department of Medicine, The Johns Hopkins University School of Medicine,
Baltimore, MD 21205, USA*
[d]*Departments of Epidemiology and Biostatistics,
Johns Hopkins Bloomberg School of Public Health, Baltimore, MD 21205, USA*
[e]*Department of Oncology, The Johns Hopkins University School of Medicine,
Baltimore, MD 21205, USA*

Evidence-based medicine (EBM) has introduced a paradigm shift in the way in which decision making is approached and clinical problems are treated in many fields of medical practice. EBM is founded on the principle that that value of health interventions should be assessed by well-designed experiments that examine the outcomes of such interventions. This is in contrast to efficacy claims grounded in physiological explanations or nonsystematic clinical observations. Although the "evidence" of EBM is generally defined in terms of outcomes-based experimentation on populations, the application of EBM to individual cases is a more difficult problem that has led to an evolution and refinement of the approach. The most recent formulation builds on the evidential foundation to incorporate a patient's clinical state and circumstances, preferences and actions, as well as the physician's clinical expertise [1].

Although EBM has now become firmly established as the desired foundation for treatment decisions in almost all medical specialties, surgery has been slower than most other medical fields to embrace it. Perhaps this can be explained by the fact that the nature of the physiological and mechanistic reasoning underlying surgical procedures often seems more accessible, and

---

* Corresponding author. 550 N. Broadway, Suite 1103, Baltimore, MD, 21205.
E-mail address: sgoodman@jhmi.edu (S.N. Goodman).

the outcomes more predictable than with many medical interventions. For example, statistical evidence from a randomized controlled trial (RCT) is not necessary to prove the value of repairing an anastomotic leak or removing an inflamed appendix. Although the value of certain surgical procedures may be self-evident, however, there are major disagreements among surgeons about the appropriateness of surgical interventions or specific techniques for many conditions. This is reflected in the considerable geographic variation in use of surgical practices for some common conditions, a variation that has led to pressure from payors and others to use evidence from clinical research to standardize procedure indications [2–5].

The demand for and use of evidence in surgical decision-making raises questions regarding what qualifies as reliable and sufficient "evidence" for a particular surgical procedure. These epistemological questions in turn create ethical tensions between surgeons' duties to foster innovation while protecting patients from harm, and between duties to benefit individual patients and populations.

This article explores several areas in which the principles of EBM, ethics, and surgical decision-making intersect. These include deciding when a surgical procedure needs formal evaluation (innovation versus experimentation), determining how that evaluation should be designed (design of surgical trials), communicating with patients about procedures supported by varying levels of evidence (informed consent), and how evidence should guide health policy and insurance coverage decisions related to surgical procedures. Those discussions are prefaced by first exploring the relationship between professional ethics and EBM, and the arguments for applying the principles of EBM to surgical practice.

Professional ethics and evidence-based medicine

The ethical duties of physicians to make treatment decisions that benefit their patients while minimizing undue risks or harms are long-established. These duties are articulated in the Hippocratic oath, and are captured in the ethical principles of "beneficence" (to promote patient well-being) and its corollary principle of "nonmaleficence" (not to harm patients) [6]. In the past century, the importance of the principle of "respect for autonomy" (respecting the self-determination of patients and encouraging participation in decision-making about treatment options) has been recognized and implemented through the process of informed consent [7–9]. The ethical principle of "justice" (fairness, including the moral imperative to allocate scarce health care resources in an equitable manner) is crucial in determining obligations to correct disparities in health care among the population [10–12]. Each of these four principles is prima facie binding; that is, they each matter in every clinical circumstance, and must be balanced against each other if they conflict [6].

The moral force of grounding treatment decisions in empirical evidence can be articulated in terms of these fundamental ethical principles. Ashcroft [13] writes that proponents of EBM "can generally be characterized as having a strong ethical sense of the importance of avoiding unnecessary harms to patients and improving health care in the interests of the general good ... . This approach had a strong ethical imperative behind it, rooted in concern to do no harm, to do one's best for one's patients, and to do so justly by eliminating waste." Physicians are entrusted with the duty to promote the well-being of patients by prescribing treatments and interventions that are on balance beneficial. Proponents of EBM contend that only well-designed clinical research can accurately quantify the risks and benefits of a procedure. Furthermore, proper informed consent can only be obtained if information about risks and benefits that is provided to patients is accurate, which often relies upon such research. Finally, evidence regarding the relative outcomes of treatments applied to well-defined groups of patients can aid policy makers in their efforts to optimally allocate resources, which can improve distributive justice in the health care system.

Although the connection between ethical surgical practice and reliable evidence may seem straightforward, there are many situations, especially those involving new surgical procedures, that present ethical challenges. How should the risks and benefits of trying a promising new intervention in a patient be weighed against the potential risks and benefits to future patient populations of not doing it as part of a formal experiment? Do surgeons have a moral obligation to subject their improved techniques to formal tests, and if so, at what stage in development of the technique? How far does respect for patients' autonomy go; can a patient demand a procedure that is unproven or even harmful; and what does a surgeon need to divulge to patients about an innovation? What evidence and how much benefit are required to justify insurance coverage or societal acceptance of a surgical procedure when health resources are limited?

Those are the kinds of questions at the interface of EBM and ethics in surgery, as well as in other medical fields. Although their resolution is beyond the scope of this piece, the authors attempt to provide a conceptual framework for their discussion.

A short history of evidence-based medicine, US regulations, and ethics

Decades before the EBM movement became formalized in the 1990s, physicians urged better evaluation of practices and better protection of patients involved in medical research [14]. Many of these arguments were rooted in concerns about professional ethics. Beginning in the early twentieth century, a small group of physicians and scientists called for therapeutic practices governed by science and not by the "idols of the marketplace or the vagaries of clinical opinion" [14]. These therapeutic reformers proclaimed that a physician who did not rely on evidence from well-designed clinical experiments was behaving unethically: "In treating patients with unproved remedies we are, whether we like it or not, experimenting on human beings, and a good experiment well reported may be more ethical and entail less shirking of duty than a poor one" [15]. The therapeutic reformers were important intellectual forerunners of EBM, who, aided by several therapeutic disasters, led the charge for establishing governmental regulations for medicinal agents. The US Food and Drug Administration (FDA) received authority for determining the safety of drugs following the elixir sulfanilamide disaster in 1938, and received the additional charge of determining efficacy as a requirement for premarket approval after narrowly averting the thalidomide disaster in the United States in the 1960s [14,16,17].

Of particular relevance to the field of surgery, United States regulations regarding medical devices emerged much later. It was only in 1976, after revelations of the thousands of women injured by the Dalkon Shield, an intrauterine birth-control device, that the FDA was authorized to require premarket approval for certain medical devices, regulating them according to level of risk [18]. In the discussion surrounding that legislation, explicit attention was paid to how device safety and efficacy could be regulated without adversely impacting innovation, an issue that arises in quite similar form in the surgical realm. Interestingly, the main assessment criteria of FDA device regulation until relatively recently was whether a medical device functioned properly and was safe, not whether it delivered therapeutic benefit. This emphasis differed from the FDA regulation of drugs and biologic agents, which have had a much longer tradition of requiring clinical trial evidence of therapeutic effect [19]. This mirrors a similar difference in philosophy between surgical and medical specialties, and may reflect a differing level of confidence in attributing the clinical effect of an intervention to a proposed mechanism.

An early prominent call for more rigorous assessment of the risks and benefits of procedures came in 1961 from an anesthesiologist at Harvard University, Henry Beecher [20]. Beecher warned of the lack of formal evaluation of many surgical procedures: "One may question the moral or ethical right to continue with casual or unplanned new surgical procedures— procedures which may encompass no more than a placebo effect—when these procedures are costly of time and money, and dangerous to health or life" [20].

In 1975, using a similar rationale, Spodik [21] called for an "FDA for surgery" that would monitor the safety and efficacy of new surgical procedures. Whereas both the FDA and institutional review boards (IRBs) have played a large oversight role in the United States in guiding the innovation and diffusion of medical therapies, development of new surgical techniques has escaped such scrutiny [22]. It has been left largely to the discretion of the field whether to designate surgical innovations as "experimental," whether patients undergoing these approaches were protected via informed consent and IRB review, and how new procedures should be evaluated and disseminated. During the mid-1990s, the American College of Surgeons formulated guidelines for the evaluation and application of emerging procedures, urging that new technologies require earlier and continued IRB review of the research protocol, along with a thorough description of informed consent of subjects [23,24]; however, these guidelines are open to interpretation and are followed at the discretion of individual surgeons. Reitsma and Moreno [22] recently claimed that the informal nature of surgical progress "pose[s] a significant ethical problem and present[s] the possibility that patients serve as unwitting subjects of research" [22].

The reasons why surgery has been reluctant to comprehensively embrace EBM for evaluation of procedures and decision-making are complex. Although caused in part by the absence of regulatory control over surgical innovation, other factors play important roles: the manner in which surgery is taught, the nature of surgical knowledge, the skill-dependence of surgery, and the unique methodological challenges for evaluating surgical procedures [22]. The traditional model for progress in surgery involves an individual surgeon developing a new procedure or incrementally improving a technique, and implementing it without formal approval by either an IRB or the patient, whose consent document may or may not reflect the novelty of the procedure. If deemed successful, the technique and clinical course of several patients is reported. As a result, the bulk of the surgical literature describing innovative procedures is comprised of case series, often uncontrolled, and many techniques disseminate into practice without formal comparison to standard or nonsurgical approaches.

The surgical field is littered with examples of operations that were developed without rigorous evaluation and disseminated widely into practice, only later to be shown in clinical trials to be ineffective or harmful. These include internal mammary artery ligation for angina [25,26], extracranial-intracranial (EC-IC) bypass to prevent the recurrence of stroke [27], gastric freezing for peptic ulcer disease [28], and more recently, arthroscopic knee surgery [29], and in certain patient subgroups, lung volume reduction surgery (LVRS) for chronic obstructive pulmonary disease (COPD) [30]. The common factors shared by such "failed" procedures are typically a plausible pathophysiologic rationale, weak early evaluation, and a strong champion.

The current effort to move away from the traditional case-series model poses several key questions. The first is when during the course of its evolution a surgical procedure should be evaluated. Answers to this question will require that a distinction be made between activities that are part of established clinical practice and those that are sufficiently innovative to require formal research. These distinctions have important ethical implications, including what to tell patients during the consent process for procedures that are considered standard practice, innovation, or experimental.

When a procedure should be formally evaluated

A major challenge for generating evidence in surgery is to decide when a procedure should be formally evaluated. A procedure may need such evaluation when there is a poor understanding of the risks and benefits of the procedure, both by itself and in relation to other therapeutic alternatives. This applies to both new procedures and those that have become common practice but remain nonvalidated; however, given the incremental development of many surgical techniques, it may be difficult to determine when a technique is sufficiently different from the standard, validated procedure to necessitate evaluation [22].

Reitsma and Moreno [22] suggest that a surgical innovation requiring formal evaluation includes "a novel procedure, a significant modification of a standard technique, a new application of or new indication for an established technique, or an alternative combination of an established technique with another therapeutic modality that was developed and tested for the first time." In a survey of surgeons who had published papers describing innovative surgeries according to this definition, Reitsma and Moreno found that 14 of 21 surgeons confirmed that their work was research, but only 6 had sought IRB approval, and only 7 mentioned the innovative nature of the procedure in the informed consent document [22]. This and other research findings have suggested that surgeons often have a poor understanding of FDA and IRB regulations for research, and raise concerns that patients are serving as unwitting subjects of research [22,31]. This has implications for the informed consent process that are discussed in a subsequent section.

The timing of evaluating rapidly evolving surgical techniques raises other practical and ethical questions. Evaluation performed too early may not test a mature procedure, and the results may be dismissed as irrelevant to practices used at the time of publication. Early evaluation also presents challenges regarding how to account for the learning curve of surgeons and their teams, because outcomes may differ between surgeons at different levels of training, and at the beginning and end of a trial. Statistical techniques are emerging to make use of such data [32].

Evaluation performed when the procedure is more mature, on the other hand, becomes difficult because widespread dissemination can render RCTs impossible or cause them to be perceived as unethical. For example, LVRS to treat COPD disseminated widely into practice before it was subject to evaluation through clinical trials. The National Emphysema Treatment Trial (NETT) trial was greatly facilitated by the US Centers for Medicaid and Medicare Services (CMS), which set a ground-breaking precedent by making involvement in an RCT a condition for reimbursement; however, in the design stage of that trial, many physicians and policy makers declared it to be unethical, based upon the fact that the procedure was widely used and their belief that its benefit was already evident [33].

Thirty years before this experience, similar debates surrounded the evaluation of coronary artery bypass grafting (CAGB). After the procedure had disseminated into practice, with many thousands of "successes" reported in large case series, some cardiologists and cardiac surgeons demanded that formal clinical trials provide statistical evidence of improved survival before endorsing the new procedure. Resistance to this was fierce, with others insisting that restoration of blood flow following CABG was sufficient visual evidence to establish its merit [34]. When these trials were finally done, they showed essentially no effect on mortality, although numerous criticisms were then aimed at the RCTs. Tales similar to the CABG story, which is told in extraordinarily rich detail by Jones [34], have been repeated in other domains and with other procedures. Experiences such as these highlight the challenge of reaching agreement about the relative merits of innovative therapies and their alternatives, and what counts as evidence—clinical, mechanistic, or statistical knowledge. The ethical acceptability of randomizing patients to alternative treatments in a research study has typically relied upon establishing equipoise, or genuine uncertainty, about the relative merits of two interventions.

These challenges suggest at least a minimum operational definition for the timing of first evaluations: when the possibility of publishing a case series is contemplated, or at the point when the surgeon who developed the procedure takes steps to disseminate the technique to others. These are implicit acknowledgments that the innovation represents a qualitative improvement, and these are key first steps in the development of generalizable knowledge. They arise at a point in the evolutionary process when either prospective cohort or randomized studies are most feasible. This comes close to the dictate by Chalmers to "randomize the first patient" [35]; however, as is discussed in the following section on choice of study design, there are multiple points in the development of a clinical procedure where it can and should be evaluated.

Choosing the most appropriate research design

The most appropriate research design is the one that is most likely to yield valid and convincing evidence to a relevant research question in a fashion both ethically permissible and acceptable to patients and physicians. Meakins [36] has observed that the surgical community is still in the process of defining its own "rules of evidence." These differ very little from traditional schemas (Table 1), but the perception of their relative value within surgery may differ somewhat from other disciplines.

The traditional "levels of evidence" in EBM, ranging lowest to highest, include expert opinion, single case reports, uncontrolled case series, case series using historical controls, observational studies, and finally RCTs. The purpose of a control or comparison group is to demonstrate the course of illness if another intervention (or nonintervention) is used. Hence, lower levels of evidence that lack controls are of limited use, given their vulnerability to bias in interpreting results. The use of historical controls runs into additional problems of bias in choosing the control group. Sometimes, however, controlled comparisons are unnecessary. One does not need such groups to tell us, for example, that a bowel obstruction must be relieved, that bleeding

Table 1
Grade of recommendations and level of evidence

Grade of recommendation	Level of evidence	Therapy/ prevention, etiology/harm	Prognosis	Diagnosis	Economic analysis
A	1a	SR of RCTs	SR of inception cohort studies, or CPG validated on a test set	SR of Level 1 diagnostic studies, or CPG validated on a test set	SR of level 1 economic studies
	1b	Individual RCT	Individual inception cohort study	Independent blind comparison of patients from appropriate spectrum, all of whom have undergone the diagnostic test and reference standard	Analysis comparing all alternative outcomes against appropriate cost measurement, and including sensitivity analysis
	1c	All or none	All of non case-series	Absolute sensitivity and specificity	Clearly as good or better, but cheaper. Clearly as bad or worse but more expensive. Clearly better or worse at the same cost
	2a	SR of cohort studies	SR of either retrospective cohort studies or untreated control groups in RCTs	SR of level >2 diagnostic studies	SR of level >2 economic studies

B				
2b	Individual cohort study	Retrospective cohort study or follow-up of untreated control patients in an RCT; or CPG not validated in a test set	Any of: -Independent blind or objective comparison -Study performed in a set of nonconsecutive patients, or confined to a narrow spectrum of study individuals (or both), all of whom have undergone both the diagnostic tests and the reference standard -A diagnostic CPG not validated in a test set	Analysis comparing a limited number of alternative outcomes against appropriate cost measurement, and including a sensitivity analysis incorporating clinically sensible variations in important variables
2c	"Outcomes" research	"Outcomes" research		
3a	SR of case-control study			
3b	Individual case-control study		Independent blind or objective comparison of an appropriate spectrum, but the reference standard was not applied to all study patients	Analysis without accurate cost measurement, but including a sensitivity analysis incorporating clinically sensible variations in important variables

(continued on next page)

Table 1 (*continued*)

Grade of recommendation	Level of evidence	Therapy/prevention, etiology/harm	Prognosis	Diagnosis	Economic analysis
C	4	Case-series (and poor quality cohort and case-control studies)	Case-series (and poor quality prognostic cohort studies)	Any of: -Reference standard was unobjective, unblinded or not independent -Positive and negative tests were verified using separate reference standards -Study was performed in an inappropriate spectrum of patients	Analysis with no sensitivity analysis
D	5	Expert opinion without explicit critical appraisal, or based on physiology, bench research, or "first principles"	Expert opinion without explicit appraisal, or based on physiology, bench research, or "first principles"	Expert opinion without explicit appraisal, or based on physiology, bench research, or "first principles"	Expert opinion without explicit appraisal, or based on economic theory

Abbreviations: CPG, clinical practice guideline; SR, systematic review.

From Meakins JL. Innovation in surgery: the rules of evidence. Am J Surg 2002;183(4):402; with permission.

must be stanched, or that the early "blue-baby" operations were successful. In such a setting, the uncontrolled clinical observations are adequate evidence. This is captured in a category of "all or none" evidence in Table 1—phenomena that we are certain will occur if not for the intervention.

But there is a continuum between "all or none" and lesser degrees of certainty. As the outcomes become slightly more distal from the intervention, the mechanisms more speculative, and the differences between alternative procedures more subtle or subjective, the need for proper controls and strong study designs increases and the weight accorded to expert opinion or mechanistic reasoning diminishes. This represents a difficult gray area because it is not always clear where the uncertainty about a clinical outcome becomes great enough to require empirical testing.

Study designs involving controlled observations, namely case-control or cohort studies, can control for relevant variables and include independent assessment of particular outcomes, greatly reduce bias, and yield reliable knowledge. Indeed, it has been argued that well-designed observational studies are best suited for evaluating that majority of surgical procedures [36,37]. Meakins [36] advocates observational studies that are prospective from the first patient, and believes that "nonrandomized trial will be the lynchpin of the knowledge development for innovative solutions to surgical disease." This may be because observational studies are able to avoid many of the methodological and ethical challenges involved in RCTs.

Randomized control trials have been considered the highest level, or gold standard, of clinical evidence, and many in the field have urged the increased use of RCTs in surgery [38,39]. Reviews of the surgical literature have concluded that there has been an underuse of RCTs [40–43], although there appears to be an increase in recent years [44,45]. The value of RCTs in both surgery and other disciplines has been repeatedly demonstrated. For example, before 1985, there were more than 200 case series published on EC-IC bypass to prevent recurrence of stroke, most of them concluding the benefits of the procedure [46]. One large RCT published in 1985 testing EC-IC bypass against medical therapy concluded that there was no reduction in the stroke rate attributable to this operation [27]. As a result, this procedure was rapidly eliminated from clinical practice as a method of stroke prevention, preventing undue harm to hundreds of future patients. The fact that a single RCT could effectively trump the evidential weight of a vast number of case series is testimony to both the value of and the need for surgical RCTs.

Despite the value of data derived from RCTs in driving medical decision making, the list of objections to randomized RCTs in surgery is quite long. It includes the inability to standardize individual surgeries and surgeons, the impracticality of locking surgeons into rigid operating protocols, problems in assessing the learning curve, the rapid evolution of technology and techniques, the inability to apply the results of clinical trials to individual surgical patients, the restricted definition of evidence these designs imply, the oversimplication of the art of surgery, difficulty with randomization in the face of strong physician or patient preferences, a jeopardized physician/patient relationship, and ethical concerns about sham surgery to control for the placebo effect [34,47–51].

These objections apply with differing force, depending on the specifics of a particular disease or surgical procedure, but rarely do they make evaluation impossible. Quite similar objections have been raised in the past and continue to be invoked to avoid randomized evaluation of both surgical and medical therapies, yet virtually all have been shown to be either baseless or solvable. The challenge is to determine both methodologically and ethically how best to address each one.

Experimentation in different stages of procedural innovation can address different questions and should have different designs. Like the models of oncologic drug development, phases of surgical evaluation could each have a design appropriate for that stage. An initial "proof of concept" evaluation would be the report of an unselected case series, which would demonstrate the technical feasibility of the operation, and perhaps a few proximal or surrogate end points. A prospective evaluation, either nonrandomized between surgeons, or randomized within a surgeon or between surgeons, with clinical outcomes, could address questions of whether the surrogate end points correlated with clinical end points, offer initial hints as to whether those clinical end points were superior in the hands of the innovator, and whether there were any predictors of which patients are likely to benefit most. Nonetheless, for observational studies, very strict controls must be maintained on recruitment and eligibility criteria to minimize selection bias and clarify the populations in whom the approach is being applied. Finally, observational and randomized studies with multiple surgeons in multiple settings could assess the outcomes of the technique when it is applied broadly, addressing the question of how it performs in more general use.

Issues related to learning curves and procedural maturation could be addressed through sequences of experiments, along with analytic methods that take into account time trends in outcome. This may render the binary question of when to evaluate a less perplexing one; procedures can and should be evaluated continually very early in their development phase, with each evaluation addressing different kinds of questions.

Choosing a control group: the ethics of sham surgery

A major ethical concern in performing RCTs is raised when the use of sham surgery is considered to control for the placebo effect. The ethical question centers on the appropriate level of harm to which research subjects can be exposed in exchange for certain benefits of generalizable knowledge and progress. There are vigorous arguments made for and against the appropriateness of sham placebo controls in surgical trials [52–54]. Several have argued that sham procedures are justified in only a few circumstances,

only after the risks have been carefully weighed against the potential benefits, and the procedure is sufficiently innocuous in nature [37,53,55,56].
Others argue that sham surgery is never ethically acceptable because the
benefits cannot outweigh the risks of an invasive procedure [52,54].

Recent RCTs that used sham surgeries have involved arthroscopic knee
surgery and fetal tissue transplantation for Parkinson disease. Those who
supported sham neurosurgery in the Parkinson's study argued that the public health benefit of guarding against a highly likely placebo effect and avoiding future unnecessary procedures outweighed the risks posed to individual
subjects [53]. Others argued that the Parkinson's study could have used alternative, less risky methods to assess the benefits and harms of fetal tissue
transplants. There is no agreement in the field as to which trial circumstances might justify the use of sham surgery, although ethical criteria have been
put forward [55].

The role of equipoise

A key ethical dimension to the problem of both the timing of surgical
evaluations and the suitability of randomized designs is captured by the concept of equipoise. The first use of the term, set forth by Charles Fried [57],
involves uncertainty on behalf an individual, informed investigator about
which of several interventions is better. The second, denoted "clinical equipoise" and proposed by Benjamin Freedman [58], requires uncertainty or
professional disagreement within the knowledgeable clinical community
about the relative merits of two therapies interventions. Freedman criticized
the original formulation as too fragile a state of uncertainty and one too dependent on the individual to be useful for a socially acceptable form of
experimentation [58].

Miller and Weijer [59] have argued that both concepts of equipoise are
necessary and address two separate moral concerns for justifying RCTs.
Fried's definition "provides a moral condition that satisfied the demands
for the continuing fiduciary relationship between physician and patient,"
whereas Freedman's "addresses the overarching need of the state to protect
its citizens from harm, and provide clear guidance to IRBs as to when a RCT
may ethically proceed" [59]. These two conceptions often collide in surgery,
however, such as when different groups of surgeons believe strongly in differing approaches. Under the principle of clinical equipoise, this is an ideal
state for the justification of an RCT, yet the requirement that individual surgeons be undecided would seem to make it either ethically or practically impossible. In these settings, a good prospective observational study may be
required to sow enough doubt to prepare the ground for an RCT.

Determining whether surgeons are in a state of clinical equipoise is difficult and varies depending upon different beliefs about what counts as evidence, as well as different interpretations of evidence [60]. As Jones [34]
notes, such disagreements "open a space for judgment and preconception,"

which may be influenced by such factors as concerns about professional authority and financial resources. In a few situations, investigators surveyed practicing clinicians to ascertain the state of practice to aid the establishment of equipoise [60]. More attention and discussion early in the development of an innovative technique is needed to address these difficult issues. For the individual surgeon, both an acknowledgment of individual preferences as well as an assessment of the larger field, combined with more open discussion with colleagues, policy members, and patients, may help guide both the timing and choice of study design.

Implications for informed consent

The ethical concerns raised by disagreements about when to evaluate procedures are linked to questions about what to tell patients who will undergo them. Standard requirements for informed consent involve explaining the proposed procedure and its risks, benefits, and alternatives [61,62]. This information must be communicated to patients in a manner in which they can understand it. In addition, patients asked to give informed consent must be positioned to make a voluntary decision [7,8]. In general, the ethical and legal standards for informed consent for clinical practice and for research are well-established.

Requirements for informed consent make it clear that meaningful informed consent for unvalidated innovations should be obtained. For operations that fall under the category of unvalidated practices or innovations, surgeons have the obligation to share what they know about the potential risks, benefits, and uncertainties of the intervention with patients. How much and which type of information is provided is ultimately up to the discretion of individual surgeons, and there are few models or standards for such interactions; however, the first, and perhaps most important step is for the surgeon to recognize and then convey to the patient the nature of the innovation and the corresponding uncertainty. The acknowledgment that a variation in a technique or procedure may have unanticipated outcomes, or risks not commensurate with benefits, is a critical step toward proper informed consent and ultimately toward proper evaluation. When innovative surgeons find themselves repeatedly describing the same uncertainties to multiple patients, this is a signal that a formal evaluation to reduce those uncertainties is required.

In the context of research, obtaining valid informed consent requires that potential subjects should understand that the goals of research are to provide generalizable knowledge, not necessarily to benefit themselves. Emphasizing the difference between the goals of established treatment and the goals of research is necessary for avoiding the therapeutic misconception and promoting informed, autonomous decisions. The term "therapeutic misconception," initially coined by Appelbaum, refers to the mistaken assumptions among research subjects that the interventions they receive during the course of research are specifically designed for their personal benefit, as they would be in clinical practice [63]. Empirical research on this phenomenon has shown that this misconception is quite common among research participants, particularly when the researcher is also a clinician who regularly treats patients [64,65]. Minimizing the therapeutic misconception in research requires careful attention to the language, manner, and context in which the goals, risks, and potential benefits are described to potential subjects.

Challenges of distributive justice

Even once the questions of when and how to evaluate innovative and nonvalidated surgical procedures are resolved, further challenges will remain in deciding what populations the experimentation should be done on, who should have access to a limited procedure, and how society should pay for such practices. That both the burdens and benefits of innovative therapy should be distributed fairly is not solved by EBM, but these problems cannot be solved without that evidence, along with detailed characterization of the populations most likely to benefit. Similarly, the problems of limited resources and funding for health care services will persist, and strengthening the evidence base for surgeries typically requires more spending rather than less. For procedures that do show benefit, the question of the incremental cost and risk for the incremental benefit arises, with concomitant societal choices forced between different procedures for different diseases. The challenge to fairly distribute health care services is not solved with evidence from clinical trials; however, such evidence can improve distributive justice by funneling resources away from expensive procedures with minimal benefit.

Summary

Evidence-based medicine, although ostensibly concerned with the research evidence underlying claims of efficacy for surgical procedures, has a direct connection with the ethics of surgical decision-making. Questions of whether new procedures should ever be performed on patients outside of a formal research protocol, what the patient should be told about the uncertainties inherent in the use of nonvalidated innovative procedures, when formal evaluation is necessary, what form that evaluation should take, and how the burdens and results of such research can be distributed fairly all involve balancing competing ethical principles. Good ethics requires good facts, and evidence from well-controlled experiments provides best information upon which to base decisions in these areas and to build ethical surgical practice.

References

[1] Haynes RB, Devereaux PJ, Guyatt GH. Clinical expertise in the era of evidence-based medicine and patient choice. ACP J Club 2002;136(2):A11–4.

[2] Dunn WR, Lyman S, Marx RG. Small area variation in orthopedics. J Knee Surg 2005; 18(1):51–6.

[3] Wennberg J, Gittelsohn A. Small area variations in health care delivery. Science 1973; 182(117):1102–8.

[4] Birkmeyer JD, Sharp SM, Finlayson SR, et al. Variation profiles of common surgical procedures. Surgery 1998;124(5):917–23.

[5] Lu-Yao G, McLerran D, Wasson JH, et al. Team TPPOR. Assessment of radical prostatectomy. Time trends, geographic variation and outcomes. JAMA 1993;269:2633–6.

[6] Beauchamp T, Childress J. Principles of biomedical ethics. New York: Oxford University Press; 2001 5th edition. 2000.

[7] Faden RR, Beauchamp TL. A history and theory of informed consent. New York: Oxford University Press; 1986.

[8] Appelbaum PS, Lidz CW, Meisel A. Informed consent: legal theory and clinical practice. New York: Oxford University Press; 1987.

[9] Emanuel EJ, Emanuel LL. Four models of the physician-patient relationship. JAMA 1992; 267(16):2221–6.

[10] Daniels N. Just health care. Cambridge (UK): Cambridge University Press; 1985.

[11] Daniels N, Sabin J. Setting limits fairly. New York: Oxford University Press; 2002.

[12] Sox H. Annals of internal medicine's Harold Sox, MD, discusses physician charter of professionalism. Interview by Brian Vastag. JAMA 2001;286(24):3065–6.

[13] Ashcroft RE. Current epistemological problems in evidence based medicine. J Med Ethics 2004;30(2):131–5.

[14] Marks HM. The progress of experiment. New York: Cambridge University Press; 1997.

[15] Mainland D. The modern method of clinical trial. Methods Med Res 1954;6:152–8.

[16] Wax PM. Elixirs, diluents, and the passage of the 1938 Federal Food, Drug and Cosmetic Act. Ann Intern Med 1995;122(6):456–61.

[17] Botting J. The history of thalidomide. Drug News Perspect 2002;15(9):604–11.

[18] Foote SB. Managing the medical arms race; innovation and public policy in the medical device industry. Oxford (UK): University of California Press, Ltd.; 1992.

[19] Merrill R. Regulation of drugs and devices: an evolution. Health Aff (Millwood) 1994;13: 47–69.

[20] Beecher H. Surgery as placebo, a quantitative study of bias. JAMA 1961;176:1102–7.

[21] Spodick D. Numerators without denominators: there is no FDA for the surgeon. JAMA 1975;232:1–32.

[22] Reitsma AM, Moreno JD. Ethical regulations for innovative surgery: the last frontier? J Am Coll Surg 2002;194(6):792–801.

[23] Surgeons ACo. Statement on emerging surgical technologies and the evaluation of credentials. Bull Am Coll Surg 1994;79:40–1.

[24] Surgeons ACo. Statement on issues to be considered before new surgical technology is applied to the care of patients. Bull Am Coll Surg 1995;80:46–7.

[25] Cobb L, Thomas G, Dillard D. An evaluation of internal-mammary-artery ligation by a double-blind technic. N Engl J Med 1959;260:1115–8.

[26] Dimond EG, Kittle F, Crockett J. Comparison of internal mammary artery ligation and sham operations for angina pectoris. Am J Cardiol 1960;5:483–6.

[27] Group TEIBS. Failure of extravranial-intracranial arterial bypass to reduce the risk of ischemic stroke: results of an internaitional randomized trial. N Engl J Med 1985;313: 1191–200.

[28] Ruffin JM, Grizzle JE, Hightower NC, et al. A co-operative double-blind evaluation of gastric "freezing" in the treatment of duodenal ulcer. N Engl J Med 1969;281(1):16–9.

[29] Moseley JB, O'Malley K, Petersen NJ, et al. A controlled trial of arthroscopic surgery for osteoarthritis of the knee. N Engl J Med 2002;347(2):81–8.

[30] The National Emphysema Treatment Trial Research Group. A randomized trial comparing lung-volume-reduction surgery with medical therapy for severe emphysema. N Engl J Med 2003;348(21):2092–102.

[31] Rutan RL, Deitch EA, Waymack JP. Academic surgeons' knowledge of Food and Drug Administration regulations for clinical trials. Arch Surg 1997;132(1):94–8.

[32] Ramsay C, Grant A, Wallace S, et al. Statistical assessment of the learning curves of health technologies. Health Technol Assess (Rockv) 2001;5:1–79.

[33] Carino T, Scheingold S, Tunis S. Using clinical trials as a condition of coverage: lessons from the National Emphysema Treatment Trial. Clin Trials 2004;1:108–21.

[34] Jones D. Visions of a cure: visualization, clinical trials, and controversies in cardiac therapeutics, 1968–1998. Isis 2000;91(3):504–41.

[35] Chalmers TC. Randomize the first patient. N Engl J Med 1977;296(2):107.

[36] Meakins JL. Innovation in surgery: the rules of evidence. Am J Surg 2002;183(4):399–405.

[37] Lilford R, Braunholtz D, Harris J, et al. Trials in surgery. Br J Surg 2004;91(1):6–16.

[38] Solomon MJ, Laxamana A, Devore L, et al. Randomized controlled trials in surgery. Surgery 1994;115(6):707–12.

[39] Solomon MJ, McLeod RS. Surgery and the randomized controlled trial: past, present, and future. Med J Aust 1998;169:380–3.

[40] Benjamin D. The efficacy of surgical treatment of cancer. Med Hypotheses 1993;40:129–38.

[41] Haines S. Randomized clinical trials in the evaluation of surgical innovation. J Neurosurg 1979;51:5–11.

[42] Gilbert J, McPeek B, Mosteller F. Statistics and ethics in surgery and anethesia. Science 1977;198:684–9.

[43] Sorenson T. Effects of treatments in clinical trials: surgery. J Surg Oncol 1993;(Suppl 3): 186–8.

[44] Hardin WD Jr, Stylianos S, Lally KP. Evidence-based practice in pediatric surgery. J Pediatr Surg 1999;34(5):908–12 [discussion: 912–13].

[45] Moss RL, Henry MC, Dimmitt RA, et al. The role of prospective randomized clinical trials in pediatric surgery: state of the art? J Pediatr Surg 2001;36(8):1182–6.

[46] Haynes RB. What kind of evidence is it that evidence-based medicine advocates want health care providers and consumers to pay attention to? BMC Health Serv Res 2002;2(1):3.

[47] Black N. Evidence-based surgery: a passing fad? World J Surg 1999;23:789–93.

[48] Cohen AM, Stavri PZ, Hersh WR. A categorization and analysis of the criticisms of evidence-based medicine. Int J Med Inform 2004;73(1):35–43.

[49] Bonchek L. Are randomized trials appropriate for evaluating new operations? N Engl J Med 1977;301:44–5.

[50] Frader J, Caniano D. Research and innovation in surgery. In: McCoullough LB, Jones JW, Brody BA, editors. Surgical ethics. New York: Oxford University Press; 1998. p. 216–41.

[51] Kadar N. The operative laparoscopy debate: technology assessment or statistical Jezebel? Biomed Pharmacother 1993;47(5):201–6.

[52] Dekkers W, Boer G. Sham neurosurgery in patients with Parkinson's disease: is it morally acceptable? J Med Ethics 2001;27(3):151–6.

[53] Albin RL. Sham surgery controls: intracerebral grafting of fetal tissue for Parkinson's disease and proposed criteria for use of sham surgery controls. J Med Ethics 2002;28(5): 322–5.

[54] Macklin R. The ethical problems with sham surgery in clinical research. N Engl J Med 1999; 341(13):992–6.

[55] Horng S, Miller FG. Ethical framework for the use of sham procedures in clinical trials. Crit Care Med 2003;31(Suppl 3):S126–30.

[56] Horng S, Miller FG. Is placebo surgery unethical? N Engl J Med 2002;347(2):137–9.

[57] Fried C. Medical experiementation: personal integrity and social policy. Amsterdam: North Holland; 1974.

[58] Freedman B. Equipoise and the ethics of clinical research. N Engl J Med 1987;317:141–5.

[59] Miller PB, Weijer C. Rehabilitating equipoise. Kennedy Inst Ethics J 2003;13(2):93–118.

[60] Tcheng JE, Madan M, O'Shea JC, et al. Ethics and equipoise: rationale for a placebo-controlled study design of platelet glycoprotein IIb/IIIa inhibition in coronary intervention. J Interv Cardiol 2003;16(2):97–105.

[61] Schloendorff v Society of New York Hospital, Court of Appeals of New York; 211 NY 125 (1914).

[62] Salgo v Leland Stanford Jr, University Board of Trustees, P2d 170 (1957).

[63] Appelbaum PS, Rothe L, Lidz C, et al. False hopes and best data. Hastings Cent Rep 1987; 17(2):20–4.

[64] Meropol NJ, Weinfurt KP, Burnett CB, et al. Perceptions of patients and physicians regarding Phase I cancer clinical trials: implications for physician-patient communication. J Clin Oncol 2003;21(13):2589–96.

[65] Weinfurt KP, Sulmasy DP, Schulman KA, et al. Patient expectations of benefit from Phase I clinical trials: linguistic considerations in diagnosing a therapeutic misconception. Theor Med Bioeth 2003;24(4):329–44.

ELSEVIER
SAUNDERS

SURGICAL
CLINICS OF
NORTH AMERICA

Surg Clin N Am 86 (2006) 169–179

Relative Contributions of Surgeons and Decision Support Systems

R. Scott Jones, MD[a,b,*], Karen Richards, BA[b], Thomas Russell, MD[b]

[a]Department of Surgery, University of Virginia Health System, PO Box 800709, Charlottesville, VA 22908–0709, USA
[b]American College of Surgeons, 633 North Saint Clair Street, Chicago, Ill 60611, USA

This article addresses the role of surgeons and decision support systems in implementing evidence-based surgery. A PubMed search to query "evidence-based surgery" revealed 2835 citations. Between 1971 and 1991, a scant one to three citations appeared annually. In about 1995, an explosive, exponential increase in references to evidence-based surgery began, and has continued to the present. This attention to evidence-based surgery followed Sackett and colleagues' [1] definition of evidence-based medicine as the conscientious, explicit, and judicious use of current best evidence in making decisions about the care of individual patients. This means application of scientifically valid patient-oriented evidence that matters (POEM) [2]. This definition also stressed the value of clinical expertise and clinical skill. The practice of evidence-based medicine must include the knowledge, experience, and skill of the physician. In the case of surgery, we cannot overlook or underestimate the value of knowledge, experience, judgment, and technical skill. The art and craft of surgery are important. Evidence-based medicine includes support of individual patient values, choices, and circumstances.

The discipline of evidence-based medicine lends itself to the care of individual patients by individual physicians, probably because it was developed by individual physicians caring for individual patients. Surgeons face the challenge of adapting to the discipline of evidence-based medicine and incorporating it into their practice. Each surgeon also treats individual patients: no two patients are the same, and no two operations are the same. Operations, although inherently variable, can be categorized. Ultimately, the universal

* Corresponding author. Division of Research and Optimal Patient Care, American College of Surgeon, 633 North Saint Clair Street, Chicago, Ill 60611.
  E-mail address: rjones@facs.org (R.S. Jones).

0039-6109/06/$ - see front matter © 2006 Elsevier Inc. All rights reserved.
doi:10.1016/j.suc.2005.10.017 *surgical.theclinics.com*

and effective application of best evidence to surgical practice may require organized systems of care. The systems will include identifying and cataloging best evidence, incorporating best evidence into the processes of care, documentation that best practices occurred, and documenting the consequences of best practices with valid outcomes data. Systems will provide the organization and infrastructure to assure best practices for all patients (Fig. 1) [3].

Problems for surgeons and evidence-based surgery

The highest level of evidence, level 1, is the systematic review of homogeneous, prospective, randomized clinical trials, followed by individual prospective randomized clinical trials with narrow confidence intervals. Level 2 evidence includes systematic reviews of cohort studies, individual cohort studies, and outcomes research. Systematic reviews of case-control studies and individual case-control studies compose level 3 evidence. Case series, poor quality cohort, and case-control studies provide level 4 evidence. The lowest level of evidence, level 5, comes from expert opinion without explicit appraisal based on physiology or bench research [4].

Since the beginning of the evidence-based medicine movement, and even before, surgeons have drawn criticism for failing to base their practices on randomized controlled trials. As recently as 1996, scrutiny of surgical journals revealed a striking majority of publications based on level 4 evidence [5]. A prospective audit of 100 consecutive patients in a general surgical/vascular unit in the United Kingdom [6] revealed that 95 received treatment based on satisfactory evidence; of those, 24 patients received treatment based on randomized controlled trial evidence, and 71 had treatment based

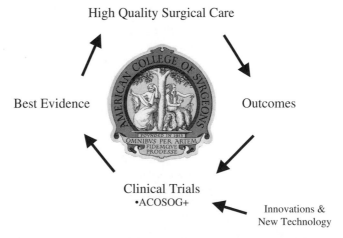

Fig. 1. High-quality surgical care depends on including best evidence into the processes of care, documenting best practices, documenting outcomes of care, and the introduction of new knowledge into practice. *From* Jones RS, Richards K. Office of Evidence-based Surgery. Bull Am Coll Surg 2003;88(4):12–21; with permission.

on other convincing evidence. The study authors went on to observe that whereas only 24% of their surgical patients' had treatment based on prospective randomized trial evidence, 50% of the internal medicine patients had treatment based on prospective randomized trials. One analysis of the illnesses and treatments most commonly encountered in general surgery found that fewer than 40% of operative treatments could be studied with prospective randomized trials [7].

Evidence-based medicine has progressed more rapidly and completely in medical disciplines than in surgical disciplines for many reasons in addition to the one cited above. Pharmaceutical companies cannot market their products without proof of safety and efficacy as required by the Food and Drug Administration (FDA). They therefore found it in their best interest to fund clinical trials, and they have done so with considerable financial investment (and return). Drug trials are relatively easy to design and conduct compared with surgical trials. The US Government barely regulates the introduction of new devices, and disregards introduction of new operations [8,9].

Surgical clinical trials are very difficult to design and conduct [7]. Variability in anatomy, pathology, surgical technique, surgical judgment, and surgical skill make standardizing operations a particular challenge, not only for clinical trial design, but for surgical quality improvement in general. Most surgeons are unwilling to participate in trials because of the paperwork, the hassle, and the discipline required. An important factor in the lack of level 1 evidence in surgical practice remains the scant support provided for clinical research in surgery. Surgical disciplines lack the trained work force, the organization and infrastructure, and funding for clinical research. National Institutes of Health (NIH) funding for clinical research in surgery lags far behind its funding for nonsurgical disciplines. For these reasons, surgeons have traditionally had less engagement with prospective randomized clinical trials than nonsurgeons. Only the National Cancer Institute's (NCI) oncology groups provide consistent support for surgical trials in the United States. Its recent addition of the American College of Surgeons Oncology Group (ACOSOG) has become an important and welcome resource for clinical research in surgery.

Although a deficiency of level 1 evidence in surgical care remains a problem, this may be improving. Perusal of surgical journals and the programs of national surgical societies reveal increasing numbers of reports of scientifically rigorous clinical trials. Some journals carry special sections focused on evidence-based surgery and endeavor to publish the results of prospective randomized trials [10], but more needs to be done.

Approaches to the problem

McCulloch [11] stated one challenge clearly and succinctly: "How do we evaluate and use an evidence base currently poor in randomized controlled trials but rich in treatments unsuitable for randomized controlled trials?"

One approach to that question is to expand the reservoir of level 1 evidence. This formidable challenge will require decades, and is reviewed in some detail elsewhere [12]. In brief, increasing level 1 evidence will require expansion of the surgical clinical scientist work force, development of the clinical research infrastructure, a change in the culture of surgery, collaboration with government and industry, and substantial increases in funding for clinical research in surgery. Surgeons (and the public) cannot wait for decades to address these matters, however; we can apply existing resources more effectively by examining our discipline carefully to identify important questions answerable by clinical trials. Surgeon/scholars can identify important questions answerable by prospective trials and work carefully to answer those questions with presently available resources. Much can be accomplished presently with scientific discipline and thoughtful scholarship.

Are surgeons making the best use of their abundant level 2, 3, and 4 data? High-quality outcomes research provides level 2 data. Our profession possesses many robust data bases, including those in institutions and those operated by professional organizations such as the Society of Thoracic Surgeons (STS), and the American College of Surgeons (ACoS), the National Cancer Database (NCDB), the National Trauma Data Bank (NTDB), and the database of the American College of Surgeons National Surgical Quality Improvement Program (ACS NSQIP). In addition, the Veterans Administration (VA) Health System maintains the Veterans Administration National Surgical Quality Improvement (VA NSQIP) database. The US Government and state governments maintain valuable clinical databases. These important resources will provide an increasing quantity and quality of level 2 evidence for incorporation into practice guidelines when level 1 evidence is lacking.

McCulloch also asserted that we need rules for determining the quality of nonrandomized studies [11]. The Cochrane Group provides a most valuable service by reviewing and assimilating level 1 evidence, making that evidence more available to clinicians in the form of guidelines. Perhaps methodologies such as the Cochrane's, directed at results of nonrandomized studies, could become a great service to surgeons and their patients. What we need is best evidence. If that happens to be level 1 evidence, that is ideal; but in the absence of level 1 evidence, we need the best evidence available. Simply put, we lack the organization for systematically determining the best evidence for directing surgical care. This does not disregard scientific discipline or rigor. We must, however, realistically strive to identify and employ the best evidence available in every instance. The leaders of surgery, using the resources of their surgical organizations, must address this important matter. Identification and application of best evidence is a professional responsibility.

Getting best evidence into practice

Accumulating and cataloging a large repository of high-quality scientific evidence will not effectively improve the quality of surgical care.

Implementing best practices will require tools or instruments for incorporating those best practices into the processes of care. The tools to serve this task include clinical guidelines, clinical pathways, algorithms, and protocols. Nugent [13] recently provided a clear, concise, and well-documented review of decision support in clinical practice, including discussion of guidelines, clinical pathways, algorithms, protocols, and risk stratification. Well-documented variations in medical and surgical practice occur in the United States [14]. This underscores the lack of professional organization and infrastructure required to identify practices based on scientific evidence, and for implementing those practices in all health care facilities throughout North America. Variability is not only a national and regional problem, but also a problem for specific diseases treated by individual surgeons. For example, McArdle and Hole [15] studied the outcomes of 645 patients who had colorectal cancer treated by 13 surgeons in one hospital. Their results revealed that: "The proportion of patients undergoing apparently curative resection varied among surgeons from 40% to 76%; overall postoperative mortality varied from 8% to 30%. After curative resection postoperative mortality varied from 0% to 20%, local recurrence from 0% to 21%, and the rate of anastigmatic leak from 0% to 25%. Survival at 10 years in patients who underwent curative resection varied from 20% to 63%, 2-year survival in those who underwent palliative resection varied from 7% to 32%, and median survival in those who underwent palliative diversion varied from 1 to 8 months" [15]. So we must address variability among surgeons within surgical systems as well as regional variability within nations. This will require defining standards of care, and implementing them by incorporating best evidence into the processes of care using guidelines.

Individual surgeons cannot identify, assimilate, and transfer into practice the large quantity of rapidly changing new knowledge and new technology required to sustain best practices. For that reason, several organizations, including the Institute of Medicine (IOM), the American Medical Association (AMA), the Canadian Medical Association (CMA), and the Agency for Health care Research and Quality (AHRQ), have established methods for developing scientifically sound clinical practice guidelines. The development of guidelines requires an extensive review of the literature, and evaluating the scientific quality of the research and the effectiveness of the studied treatment. Expert panels review the guidelines, then submit them to peer review before publication. These carefully prepared guidelines can provide surgeons with rationales and strategies for making treatment decisions. Implementation of guidelines can improve the processes of care in 90% of cases, and can improve outcomes in 20% of cases [16]. Implementation becomes an important issue for the effectiveness of guidelines in improving clinical care.

Mere publication in books and journals will not incorporate clinical guidelines into practice effectively [17]. Organizations such as the Cochrane Group and the Internet have substantially enhanced the applicability of guidelines. Local opinion leaders or the professional leadership in health systems provide the most effective means for improving the compliance with clinical practice guidelines to date [18]. Promoting the use of clinical practice guidelines is an excellent opportunity and responsibility for professional organizations [17].

Whereas clinical guidelines define ideal treatment strategies for particular diseases, clinical pathways delineate the optimal sequence of timing of interventions for diagnoses and procedures. Clinical pathways delineate the steps and processes of care to implement the strategy defined in the clinical guideline. Multidisciplinary teams organize, implement, and carry out all of the components of the pathways, including clinical assessments, routine interventions, diagnostic procedures, medications, activities, nutritional concerns, consultations, rehabilitation services, social services, pastoral care, patient and family education, discharge planning, and follow-up. The team defines the expected sequence of events for an uncomplicated disease course to detect and correct departures from the expected as early as possible. Pathways can promote communication, teamwork and promote safety.

Algorithms, flow diagrams with branching-logic pathways, introduce flexibility within clinical pathways. Diagnostic algorithms sort diagnostic functions within the pathway, and management algorithms add specific treatments based on specific clinical criteria. For example, an algorithm for the diagnosis and treatment of atrial fibrillation can standardize the care of an important subset of patients. Protocols are individual treatment plans applied within clinical pathways. Protocols for early postoperative endotracheal extubation, insulin administration for diabetics, and anticoagulation administration provide examples.

Surgeons, working through their professional societies, will foster the development of systems and infrastructure to recognize and incorporate best evidence into the standard of surgical care. After establishing processes, the systems have the responsibility of monitoring compliance with best practices. How often do patients receive the established processes of care? Quality indicators can verify compliance with established care processes. Examples include: What percent of patients received preoperative prophylactic antibiotics when indicated?; What percent of patients received perioperative beta blockers when indicated?; What percent of patients received perioperative prophylaxis for deep venous thrombosis?; What percent of patients had their surgical site marked preoperatively?; What percent of patients had correct discharge instructions? Surgeons can contribute to the practice of evidence-based surgery by documenting that evidence-based care actually occurred in every patient encounter.

Outcomes

How do surgeons know if their evidence-based processes of care work? They measure their outcomes. Nonsurgeons have more practices based on level 1 evidence than surgeons, and a greater repository of level 1 evidence than surgeons. Nonsurgeons have limited opportunity for monitoring or quantifying outcomes of their care. Therefore, nonsurgeons focus on the processes of care. Surgeons have fewer practices bases on level 1 evidence and a small repository of level 1 evidence. Surgeons have abundant opportunities for quantifying their outcomes. Surgeons have preoperative data to predict postoperative outcome. So, nonsurgeons focus attention to processes of care, whereas surgeons tend to focus on outcomes. In reality, quality improvement in surgery requires attention to processes and outcomes.

In addition to evaluating the effectiveness of the processes of care, scrutiny of outcomes can monitor the consequences of the introduction of new technology or new standards. For example, review of a New York state database detected an increase in bile duct injuries following the introduction of laparoscopic cholecystectomy [19]. Outcome databases are an essential element of evidence-based surgery. Many institutions maintain databases, including surgical outcomes data: among them are the US Government, many states, insurance corporations, and other corporations such as the University Health System Consortium.

For surgeons to fulfill their role in the practice of evidence-based surgery they must own, operate, design, and manage surgical outcome databases. Administrative databases lack the clinical specificity required for effective surgical quality improvement. For many years, surgeons have recognized the importance of outcomes data. In 1990, the VA introduced the National Surgical Quality Improvement Program (NSQIP). This became the first peer-controlled, reliable, biostatistically rigorous, validated, risk-adjusted quality improvement program in surgery [20]. The NSQIP served very well, and for that reason in 2000 the VA and the ACoS began collaboration to employ the NSQIP in the private sector by studying general and vascular surgery. This collaboration produced the ACS NSQIP, now available to private hospitals [21].

The ACS NSQIP depends on a database that includes preoperative, intraoperative, and 30-day postoperative data. Multiple logistic regressions identify the significant risk factors for morbidity and mortality, allowing prediction of expected outcomes. Comparing the expected outcome to the observed outcomes (O/E ratio) provides quantification of surgical quality and permits valid comparisons of outcomes between hospitals.

The ACS NSQIP requires a surgeon leader in each participating hospital. A trained, dedicated surgical clinical nurse reviewer (SCNR) collects and submits the required data. A carefully defined data collection process provides a statistically valid sample of each hospital's operations. The effectiveness of the program depends on the accuracy, quality, and reliability of the submitted data. The SCNRs receive initial and continuing training, as well as annual quality evaluation [20].

The ACS NSQIP maintains a Web site for surgeons to examine their data and compare their performance with the averages of the hospitals in the program. The Web site provides to participants continuously updated clinical performance improvement reports, online reports and benchmarking, postoperative occurrence (complication) reports, wound class reports, preoperative risk factors reports, mortality reports, length of stay reports, procedure reports, and surgical performance measures reports.

In addition, each hospital receives a semiannual written report with an analysis of its outcomes and a confidential comparison with all other hospitals in the program.

In 1986 the ACoS, the American Cancer Society (ACS), and the Commission on Cancer (CoC) developed the NCDB, which currently includes 16 million cancer patient records. More recently, the ACoS Committee on Trauma (CoT) founded the NTDB, which currently has records on 1.5 million trauma victims. The STS operates a robust and effective database on thoracic and cardiovascular surgery. More recently, with a grant from the AHRQ, the VA collaborated with the ACoS to move the NSQIP into the private sector. The Society of American Gastrointestinal Endoscopic Surgeons (SAGES) operates an effective database on gastrointestinal surgery.

Surgeons currently possess effective databases, but need additional resources for additional surgical specialties. Also, surgeons need to learn how to use the existing databases more effectively in research, but especially for purposes of quality improvement and as tools for implementing evidence-based surgery.

American College of Surgeons centers for surgical care: development of care systems

We possess an abundant repository of evidence for surgical care. Various authors have prepared approximately 3000 clinical guidelines of variable quality. Level 1 evidence supports many of those guidelines. A small fraction of level 1 guidelines relate to surgical care, but the important and immediate point is to translate the evidence base into processes of care. Books, journals, the Internet, and dedicated surgeon advocates cannot incorporate best evidence into the processes of care with the effectiveness required [17]. So if we consider evidence-based surgery seriously, we must address the important question of implementation; and to address implementation, we must develop systems for providing care. Who bears the responsibility for organizing systems of surgical care? The authors quote Paul Starr: "A profession, sociologists have suggested, is an occupation that regulates itself through systematic, required training and collegial discipline; that has a base in technical, specialized knowledge; and that has a service rather than a profit orientation, enshrined in its code of ethics" [22]. Perhaps the surgical profession has the responsibility for establishing systems to implement evidence-based practice [17]. Achieving safe, high quality, evidence-based surgical care will require collaborative leadership among all of the surgical professional organizations. A professionally organized system for surgical care will set evidence-based standards, implement evidence-based processes of care, document the application of evidence-based standards of care, and document the outcomes of care. Examples of such systems currently exist.

The AcoS, in partnership with the ACS and the Commission on Cancer, currently approve and verify over 1400 cancer centers. The approved centers must adhere to 36 standards, must have specified organization and infrastructure, must employ guidelines, must implement a quality improvement program, and must monitor outcomes using the NCDB. The Cancer Center Approvals Program provides a prototype organization for promoting evidence-based surgery by implementing guidelines, clinical pathways, outcome measurement, and the introduction of new knowledge. The Cancer Center Approvals Program sets standards, implements the application of standards, and monitors the application of the standards. To maintain approval, cancer centers must undergo site visits every 3 years.

The ACoS CoT has established approximately 200 trauma centers. These trauma programs are analogous to the cancer programs. The CoT sets standards, stipulates required human and physical resources, defines processes of care, measures outcomes with the NTDB, and facilitates the introduction of new technology. The CoT instituted the Advanced Trauma Life Support System (ATLS), an excellent example of a well-organized clinical pathway. The ATLS system establishes a protocol for the resuscitation of injury victims, minimizing variability in the care of seriously injured patients in the emergency department.

Recognizing the value of the cancer programs and trauma programs, the regents of the ACoS instructed the staff to develop additional center programs using those established principles, outlined in Box 1 . They recognize

---

Box 1. American College of Surgeons centers

Organization and leadership

Resource Standards

Physical resources
Human resources
   Credentialing standards
Process of care standards
   Evidence-based guidelines
   Clinical pathways
   Algorithms
   Protocols
Outcomes
Verification

the urgent and pressing need to extend these established quality improvement practices beyond trauma and cancer into other disciplines of surgical care, and instructed the college staff to develop additional types of centers to promote evidence-based disease management. Cancer centers and trauma centers address disciplines. Future ACoS centers will address the management of diseases and credentialing surgeons. The center designation will be entirely voluntary, and will include hospitals and outpatient facilities.

Only facilities recognized by the Joint Commission for Accreditation of Health care Organizations, American Osteopathic Association, or the American Association for Accrediting Ambulatory Health Care Centers can participate in the program. Each center addressing a specific disease or operation, such as obesity and bariatric surgery, will have a surgeon leader, and a designated health care professional to organize and supervise the program and the associated personnel. The facilities leadership will recognize and support the center program, providing the stipulated resources required. The center will require disease- or procedure-related equipment, transportation, ward care equipment and furniture, operating room equipment, surgical intensive care unit equipment, imaging resources, and endoscopy resources. Proper surgical care requires multidisciplinary support, including multiple medical specialties, nursing, allied health professions, and administrative support. ACoS Centers will stipulate the human resources required for disease-specific centers. Box 1, above, shows the template for resources in the proposed centers. Some of these require additional comment. "Human resources" involves assembling the necessary multidisciplinary teams, including medical specialists, nurses, allied health professionals, and administrative staff where necessary. Center-designated surgeons will have appropriate licensure, American Board of Medical Specialties certification, procedure-specific training, procedure volume standards, continuing medical education requirements, and documentation of clinical outcomes. The centers will establish evidence-based processes of care aligned with clinical practice guidelines and clinical pathways. Centers will have the option of monitoring outcomes using the ACS NSQIP database or an ACoS procedure-specific database. Enrollment in ACoS Centers will require an initial site visit. Continuing participation will require an annual written status report and a site visit every 3 years. The annual standardized written status report will include assessment of morbidity and mortality outcomes, status of staffing, and review of resources available for the year ended. The triannual site visits will include review of a previsit questionnaire and checklist, interviews with center leaders, inspection of relevant facilities, review of medical records, and review of the outcomes database with the care team.

Summary

Surgeons bear responsibilities to individual patients and to the public to provide effective, efficient, and professional care for all. Efficacies, low mortality, low morbidity, and prompt and courteous service should characterize that care. Those goals can be accomplished by establishing systems, organization, and infrastructure for incorporating best evidence into the processes of care, compliance with best practices, documentation of compliance with best practices, and documenting the outcomes of care with reliable data.

References

[1] Sackett DL, Straus SE, Richardson WS, et al. Evidence-based medicine. 2nd edition. Toronto (Canada): Churchill Livingstone; 2000.

[2] Slawson DC, Shaugnessy AF, Bennet JH. Becoming a medical information master: feeling good about not knowing everything. J Fam Pract 1994;38:505–13.

[3] Jones RS, Richards K. Office of evidence-based surgery. Bull Am Coll Surg 2003;88(4):12–21.

[4] Centers for evidence-based medicine. Oxford. Available at: http://www.cebm.net. Accessed December 12, 2005.

[5] Horton R. Surgical research or comic opera, questions but few answers. Lancet 1996;347: 984–5.

[6] Howes N, Chagla L, Thorpe M, McCulloch P. Surgical practice is evidence-based. Br J Surg 1997;84:1220–3.

[7] McLeod RS, Wright JG, Solomon MJ, Hu X, et al. Randomized controlled trials in surgery: issues and problems. Surgery 1996;119:483–6.

[8] Reitsma AM, Moreno JD. Ethical regulations for innovative surgery: the last frontier? J Am Coll Surg 2002;194(6):792–801.

[9] Strasberg S, Ludbrook PA. Who oversees innovative practice? Is there a structure that meets the monitoring needs of new techniques? J Am Coll Surg 2003;196(6):938–48.

[10] Eberlein T. Evidence-based surgery. J Am Coll Surg 2005;200(6):A37–40.

[11] McCulloch P. Evidence-based general surgery. 1999.

[12] Jones RS, Debas IIT. Research: a vital component of optimal patient care in the United States. Ann Surg 2004;240(4):573–7.

[13] Nugent W. Decision support in clinical practice: guidelines, pathways, algorithms, protocols, and risk stratification. In: Manuel BM NP, editor. Surgical patient safety: essential information for surgeons in today's environment. Chicago: American College of Surgeons; 2004.

[14] Wenenberg J. The Dartmouth atlas of health care. Chicago: American Hospital Publishing, Inc.; 1998.

[15] McArdle CS, Hole D. Impact of variability among surgeons on post operative morbidity and mortality and ultimate survival. BMJ 1991;302:1501–5.

[16] Goldfarb S. The utility of decision support clinical guidelines, and financial incentives as tools to achieve improved clinical performance. Jt Comm J Qual Improv 1999;25:137–44.

[17] Eagle KA, Lee TH, Brennan TA, et al. Guideline implementation. J Am Coll Cardiol 1997;29:1141–8.

[18] Wise CG, Billi JE. A model for practice guideline adaptation and implementation: empowerment of the physician. Jt Comm J Qual Improv 1995;21:465–76.

[19] Bernard HR, Hartman TW. Complications after laparoscopic surgery. Am J Surg 1993; 165:533–5.

[20] Khuri SF, Daley J, Henderson WC. The comparative assessment and improvement of quality of surgical care in the Department of Veterans Affairs. Arch Surg 2002;137:20–7.

[21] Fink AS, Campbell DA, Mentzer RM. The National Surgical Quality Improvement Program in non-Veterans Administration hospitals. Ann Surg 2002;236:344–54.

[22] Starr P. The social transformation of American medicine. Basic Books; 1982.

SURGICAL
CLINICS OF
NORTH AMERICA

Surg Clin N Am 86 (2006) 181–192

Developing Skills for Evidence-Based Surgery: Ensuring that Patients Make Informed Decisions

Albert G. Mulley, Jr, MD[a,b,*]

[a]*General Medicine Division and Medical Practice Evaluation Center,
Massachusetts General Hospital, 50 Staniford Street, Suite 900, Boston, MA 02114, USA*
[b]*Harvard Medical School, 50 Staniford Street, 9-962, Boston, MA 02114, USA*

Some surgical decisions are straightforward. The diagnosis is indisputable. All would agree that the anticipated outcome in the absence of the intervention is dire, and surgery is known to be highly effective in preventing the dire outcome and to confer minimal risk of death or serious complications. Such is the situation in the case of ruptured abdominal viscous or certain traumatic injuries. There may be a real sense of urgency, because delay may diminish the effectiveness of surgery. The patient or family members should be as well-informed as possible about the case for surgery, but there should be little need for detailed explanation or negotiation.

Other surgical decisions are more complex. There may be a high degree of uncertainty about the effectiveness of surgery compared with alternative treatments. There may be significant disagreement among different people about the impact of the relevant health states—both indications for and outcomes of treatment—on quality of life. Making good decisions in the face of such uncertainty and disagreement requires informing patients about the options and likely outcomes of each choice, but this can be difficult and time consuming. It also requires helping patients to understand how they feel about the relevant health states—both those they have experienced and those they haven't. This too can be a challenge. Neither doctor nor patient can make a good decision alone. Even when working well together,

This work was supported by funding from the Foundation for Informed Medical Decision Making. Dr. Mulley receives royalties from Health Dialog, Inc.

* General Medicine Division, Massachusetts General Hospital, 50 Staniford Street, Suite 900, Boston, MA 02114.

E-mail address: amulley@partners.org

doi:10.1016/j.suc.2005.11.001
surgical.theclinics.com

doctor and patient can benefit from system support that facilitates communication of information and clarifies patients' values.

There is ample evidence to suggest that the challenge of making complex surgical decisions is not being fully met [1,2]. In one systematic review of more than 1000 encounters between patients and their primary care providers or surgeons [3], fewer than 1% of complex decisions could be considered completely informed. In order for progress to be made, surgeons and their clinical colleagues will have to recognize obstacles to effective communication of both information and vicarious experience to patients. Patients and family members will have to develop a clearer understanding of their roles in decision making. And perhaps most importantly, policy makers will have to find ways to invest in the systems support, including incentives and rewards, for doctors and patients to work more effectively together as collaborators [2].

All of this will be necessary to measurably improve the quality of many common surgical decisions. Relevant professional knowledge will have to be made available to and understood by the patient or family member, so that no potentially fateful decision is made in the face of avoidable ignorance. Decisions should reflect what patients care most about as they anticipate likely outcomes of alternative treatment choices. Put differently, surgeons should work to minimize unwarranted variation in the use and interpretation of evidence in the process of decision-making. And they should elicit and respect the different preferences of different patients and thereby personalize the treatment choices [2]. This approach to the surgeon's role in ensuring that patients make informed decisions that are right for them can best be appreciated with an understanding of practice variation and responses to it over the past 2 decades.

Practice variation and implications for informed surgical decisions

In 1982, in the New England Journal of Medicine, McPherson and colleagues [4] published an analysis of geographic variation in rates of seven surgical procedures in their respective countries—England, Norway, and the United States—that raised serious questions about the quality of surgical decision-making. There was consistency among the three countries in the degree of variability for procedures. Tonsillectomy, hemorrhoidectomy, hysterectomy, and prostatectomy varied more among geographic areas than appendectomy, hernia repair, or cholecystectomy. Degree of variation was more characteristic of the procedure than of the country, suggesting that it reflected differences in doctors' beliefs about the value of procedures in meeting patients needs rather than differences in ways of organizing or paying for care. Wennberg and coworkers [5] called this the "professional uncertainty hypothesis."

It was not the first time that such variations had been documented. Wennberg had previously published similar findings from New England states, and Glover had done so for the midlands of England in 1938, a decade before the establishment of Britain's National Health Service [5]. The earlier studies had attracted little attention from surgeons, patients, or policy makers. But in 1982, the cost and quality implications of these findings were too great to be ignored. Other investigators replicated Wennberg's findings in larger populations. Interdisciplinary collaborations were formed to better understand variation and to develop constructive responses. The overall impact during the ensuing decade was far more attention to surgical decision-making, including the quality of supporting evidence and the importance of patients' preferences regarding trade-offs between benefits and harms of surgical and nonsurgical approaches to common clinical conditions.

Professional uncertainty and unwarranted variation

The professional uncertainty hypothesis raised serious challenges regarding the clinical relevance of professional knowledge base, and the skill with which that knowledge was managed for use in clinical decision-making [5]. It was recognized that professional uncertainty might reflect real limits of medical knowledge when the relevant research has not been conducted, as was the case for many of the most common surgical procedures that exhibited marked variation. At the time the McPherson and colleagues paper [4] was published, there had been no randomized trials of tonsillectomy, hemorrhoidectomy, hysterectomy, or prostatectomy. But professional uncertainty might also result from inadequate information on the part of some doctors when that information is available to others. The former has been referred to as collective professional uncertainty, the latter as individual professional uncertainty [6]. It is important to make this distinction, because these problems have different solutions: more relevant research in the first case, and more effective knowledge management and dissemination in the second [1,6]. The last 2 decades have seen great strides in both areas, directed at reducing the unwarranted variation in clinical practices seen when local conventional wisdom reflects unfounded enthusiasm or local capacity to perform procedures rather than what the evidence indicates about effectiveness. Perhaps most notable is the remarkable collection of systematic reviews of randomized trials, many addressing the effectiveness of surgical interventions, produced by the Cochrane Collaboration.

Other approaches proved to be less constructive. Consensus methods were used to develop "appropiateness criteria" that were then used by health plans and payers to develop preauthorization criteria and second-opinion programs. Such programs had little or no effect on procedure rates, and were generally viewed by surgeons and patients alike as intrusions in the doctor-patient relationship. Clinicians also argued that such approaches did not sufficiently account for important clinical differences among patients.

Patient preferences and warranted variation

Practice variation measured from case to case may reflect differences in valuations made by different people (or for different people) for the same health state. When the purpose of a surgical procedure is to reduce bothersome symptoms, the surgical indication depends directly on just how bothered the particular patient is, and how bothered he or she would be by any symptoms related to a complication or side effect of the surgery. Examples of these "preference-sensitive" surgical decisions include hysterectomy for pelvic pain or abnormal vaginal bleeding, back surgery for back or leg pain attributable to herniated lumbar disc or spinal stenosis, or hip or knee replacement for the pain of osteoarthritis. The construct of preference-sensitive surgical decisions was first described in the context of transurethral resection of the prostate (TURP) as treatment for men who have urinary dysfunction attributable to benign prostatic hyperplasia (BPH) [7–9]. That case study remains instructive, especially for the surgeon whose goal is to work with patients to make informed decisions.

Benign prostatic hyperplasia and the importance of patients' preferences

BPH affects the majority of older men, producing some degree of urinary dysfunction. Endoscopic approaches to reduce obstruction to urinary flow by removing prostatic tissue evolved during the early part of the twentieth century. From the perspective of surgical investigators, there was sufficient evident effect on urinary flow rates, post-void residual urine volume, and other physiologic measures to justify use of TURP for decades before the first randomized trial was reported in 1995 [10]. Nearly a decade before, Barry and colleagues [11] had shown that the physiologic measures used in the earlier observational studies were poorly correlated with the lower urinary tract symptoms of most concern to patients. With the American Urological Association (AUA) symptom index, and later the International Prostate Symptom Score (IPSS), investigators and clinicians were able to shift the focus of effectiveness measures to symptom reduction [12,13].

Barry and colleagues also discovered that men who have the same symptom score might be more bothered or less bothered by the same level of symptoms [7,8]. The practical implication of this finding for urologists was the necessity of carefully inquiring of patients not just about frequency and severity of urinary symptoms, but also about the degree of bother. The answer to the question, "How much are you bothered by your symptoms?" became the key data point in determining whether or not surgery was indicated [12,13]. Corollary questions, such as, "Do your symptoms keep you from doing anything that is important to you or that you especially enjoy, and thereby decrease the quality of your life?" can help the patient clarify his values and be thoughtful about his response regarding bother.

Another important finding in the work by Barry and coworkers was the great collective professional uncertainty, often not expressed, about the natural history of BPH. In the absence of good longitudinal studies, doctors varied widely in their estimates of the likelihood of complicating events such as acute urinary retention, and could only hypothesize about the inevitability or pace of symptom progression [9,14]. The question, "What happens if I do nothing but watchfully wait, or monitor my condition?" was rarely asked by patients, and because of the profound collective professional uncertainty, the answers were rarely volunteered by clinicians. But without consideration of the natural history of BPH, estimation of the net effects of intervention was impossible for patients or their clinicians.

The bother of urinary symptoms, now and in the future, and how it might be ameliorated by surgical intervention were not the only relevant outcomes. For the man who chooses surgery, there is a high probability of symptom relief, but also a significant probability of surgical complications. For some men, surgery could make urinary symptoms worse; permanent post-surgical urinary dysfunction such as persistent incontinence is rare, but it does occur. Surgical complications can lead to death in the perioperative period. Probabilities are low for most men, but increase with age or comorbidities such as heart disease or lung disease.

Most men who are treated with traditional TURP experience sexual dysfunction in the form of retrograde ejaculation. Men vary significantly in their subjective response to this health state [7,8]. Some accommodate to the difference in the sexual experience quickly and enjoy sex as much as or more than ever. Others do not accommodate and are so troubled that they stop having sex, despite unimpaired erectile function. Here the task of informing the patient is complex. He should understand not only the likelihood of retrograde ejaculation as a consequence of surgical intervention—its usual lack of relationship to erectile function, its implications for fathering children—but also what it will mean to him personally. If he imagines its impact incorrectly, underestimating or overestimating any decrement in the quality of sexual experience, he will make a less than optimal decision [15].

The clinician may be able to help patients imagine new health states more accurately than they can alone, and predict the impact on quality of life, by virtue of the vicarious experience they have gained with other patients who have experienced those states. Sometimes conversations with experienced patients can be useful for the patient currently confronting the choice. But there is great potential for bias when clinicians and experienced patients do not recognize the range of subjective responses to the same health state, and that it is the personal response of the patient facing the decision that is crucial to the decision making process. This approach to ensuring that patients make informed decisions can be summarized by enumerating just a few questions that the clinician can ask about both patient knowledge and patient values. These are listed in Box 1.

Box 1. Clinician questions about patient knowledge and values concerning benign prostatic hyperplasia

Ensuring essential knowledge
Do you know what options you have for treatment?
Do you understand what will happen if you choose no treatment?
Do you understand the probability and degree of symptom relief
    that you can expect with the different treatment options?
Do you understand the probability and degree of sexual function
    that you can expect with the treatment options?

Facilitating clarification of values
How bothered are you by your urinary symptoms?
What is it that you can't do because of your urinary symptoms
    that you miss the most?
How much symptom relief is necessary to let you do what you
    miss doing?
What risk are you willing to accept to obtain that?
How bothered are you by the prospect of sexual dysfunction,
    especially those that occur commonly with some treatment
    options (eg, retrograde ejaculation)?

Tools have been developed to facilitate this approach to supporting patients in making informed decisions, providing answers to the essential knowledge questions and tasks or the experience of prior patients to help clarify values. Some of these tools are simple pamphlets or brochures with worksheets. Others use computer technology, video, and other media to provide information and vicarious patient experience. Such decision aids can be constructed to fully reflect the range of patients' responses to the same outcomes, with descriptions from multiple experienced patients to reflect that range [16–18]. Decision aids can also be used to tailor information to the clinical circumstances of the individual patient. Complication and mortality rates can be estimated in light of the particular patient's age, disease severity, and comorbidity. Graphical presentations can be used to provide a balanced framing of good and bad outcomes, and their distribution over time [19–23].

When such decision aids are used, studies have shown that they increase patients' knowledge of therapeutic options and likely outcomes, to a level comparable to that of urology nurses in the case of BPH [24]. There is also evidence to suggest that they help patients to clarify their preferences when the decision requires trade-offs related to personal views about quality of life [17,18]. In one study [25], the degree of bother with urinary dysfunction and the predicted bother with future sexual dysfunction were the most important predictors of treatment choice for men who had BPH. Men who were very bothered by their symptoms—whether the symptom score could be characterized as mild, moderate, or severe—were seven times more likely to have surgery than men who were not bothered very much by symptoms. Men who predicted that they would be very bothered by any sexual dysfunction that followed surgery were one fifth as likely to undergo TURP as men who predicted that they would not be very bothered by changes in sexual function [25]. The use of such an approach has been well-received by patients in the United Kingdom and Canada as well as the United States [26,27]. Although some surgeons have incorporated decision aids into their practices, many do not recognize the need to do so, and their use is not widespread.

Applying the lessons learned in benign prostatic hyperplasia more broadly

The potential for this approach to decision-making is not limited to BPH. Rather it applies to all surgical decisions made in the face of uncertainty with potential disagreement about the impact of relative outcomes. Some of these decisions and conditions have structures very similar to the BPH decision. For example, treatment of benign uterine conditions with hysterectomy has a high probability of relieving symptoms, but may be followed by some forms of sexual dysfunction in some women. How bothered is the patient at hand by her symptoms, and how would she feel about any decrease in libido or change in her experience of sexual activity? When the bothersome symptom is excessive bleeding due to fibroids, an important difference between this situation and the predicament of the man who has BPH is that bleeding is likely to stop when the patient reaches menopause, making a strategy of nonsurgical treatment attractive to ameliorate symptoms during the interval period. Though symptoms attributable to BPH wax and wane on a weekly or daily basis, the general tendency is for them to increase over time. The question for the woman who has uterine bleeding is, "Can I be patient enough to let symptoms resolve over time without surgery?" For the man who has lower urinary tract symptoms and BPH, it is, "Have I reached the threshold beyond which the bother of symptoms justifies the risks and side effects of surgery?"

Patients who have back pain and leg pain attributable to anatomic problems amenable to surgery face similar questions. Patients who have a clear anatomic explanation for their symptoms in the form of a herniated lumbar disk are likely to experience symptom relief sooner rather than later with surgery. But over time, there is no difference in prevalence of pain following either surgical or nonsurgical treatment. As always, surgery entails some risks, including that of failed back surgery syndrome with persistent, refractory back pain. So again, the question for many patients is, "Can I be patient enough to let symptoms resolve over time without surgery and thereby avoid its risks?" Pain associated with spinal stenosis is not likely to resolve over time. Like the symptoms of BPH, it is likely to wax and wane, but generally and gradually progress over time. The same is true for either hip or knee pain attributable to osteoarthritis. Each patient will have his or her own threshold for symptoms' negative impact on quality of life that justifies the risks of surgery.

Informing patients about risks of death and other bad outcomes

For the examples used so far, death is not a near-term consequence of the condition itself. It becomes a concern with the surgery option because of the small but real probability of operative complication and resulting mortality. As noted, patients will have different responses to these small risks and different thresholds for distinguishing between a risk that is acceptable to them from one that is unacceptable. Accurate estimation of these risks and their communication can be a challenge. Again, carefully designed decision aids, especially those that allow for risk estimates tailored to the particular patient's clinical circumstances, can help in overcoming these obstacles [19–23].

Other conditions do confer risk of death, and the purpose of surgery may be to reduce mortality risk or at least delay death, as is the case with most cancer surgery. As noted at the outset, when surgery is known to be effective at preventing an outcome about which there is little or no disagreement, decisions can be straightforward. But when effectiveness is uncertain, when decrease in risk is marginal, or when different surgical options involve a trade-off between lower risk of bad outcomes in the future but greater morbidity in the near term, the decisions and the patients' information needs are complex. The classic example of this kind of decision focused on the trade-off between speech and survival prospects for patients who had laryngeal cancer. The key finding was that different individuals saw the trade-offs differently, and as a result preferred different treatment choices [28].

Many patients confronted with surgical decisions aimed at reducing risk of death present with minimal or no symptoms. This is the case for many patients newly diagnosed with the most common cancers—cancer of the breast, prostate, colon, and lung. Quality of life is affected by the diagnosis and what it portends for the future. Many such patients go from feeling perfectly well at one moment to "terminally ill" the next. They feel more vulnerable than ever before. Information about the future may imply responsibility for decision-making that they do not want, at least at the moment. Often, emotional support from family and friends as well as professionals is the first priority as they try to sort through the emotions. There is often a sense of urgency that may or may not be real. It rarely is, for instance, in the case of either prostate cancer or breast cancer. In such cases, the clinician can help prepare the patient for informed decision-making by addressing emotional issues, helping to identify sources of support, and relieving any false sense of urgency [29].

Does the evidence provide answers to patients' most pressing questions?

Inattention to what matters most to patients, and the disagreement among patients about the quality-of-life impact of different health states, can lead to an evidence base that leaves patients' most pressing questions unanswered. One example of this phenomenon can be found in those studies that determined the equivalence of mastectomy versus lumpectomy followed by radiation for women who had early-stage breast cancer. The early trials did indeed determine survival equivalence, but the way results were reported created lasting confusion about the equivalence with regard to breast cancer recurrence. The authors of one study [30] excluded ipsilateral in-breast recurrences when reporting equivalent disease-free survival, and later reported [31] that such recurrences occurred at a rate of greater than 1% per year for a 10-year period. A subsequent trial addressing the same question [32] emphasized recurrence rates after "censoring" ipsilateral, in-breast recurrences that were susceptible to salvage mastectomy. In neither case was the intent to mislead. Rather, there was an underlying assumption about the relative importance of different outcomes that determined what was reported. It is now widely recognized that some women are sanguine about the risk of future ipsilateral, in-breast recurrence, but others dread that prospect. Recognition of these differences would have dictated more careful measurement and reporting of the outcome, allowing more informed decisions about treatment choice tailored to the personal concerns of individual patients [1].

In some areas, important patient concerns were not addressed during the conduct of research that was highly influential in shaping indications for surgery because of the specialized interests and research focus of specialist investigators. Coronary artery bypass graft (CABG) was first performed in 1967 and was subsequently subjected to seven randomized trials, including more than 2500 participants. None of the participants was older than 65 years of age. Because the trials were conducted among younger patients by cardiologists and cardiac surgeons, little attention was given to the neuropsychiatric complications of surgery. It was not until the early 1990s, after aggressive indications for CABG among older patients were already well established, that the high risk of stroke and cognitive dysfunction in this population was recognized [1].

Integrating decision support and clinical trials to improve relevant knowledge

Approaches to collecting evidence that is relevant to patients, and that simultaneously supports the quality of patients' decisions, have been developed and implemented. In these "preference trials," patients are fully informed about treatment options and probabilities of outcomes, and are provided with support to help them clarify their valuations with a decision aid, health coach, or both. Those who prefer surgical treatment undergo surgery. Those whose prefer to avoid surgery undergo nonsurgical therapy. And those who find that each treatment approach is equally attractive (or unattractive) are offered randomization. All four treatment groups—preferred surgery, preferred nonsurgical treatment, randomized to surgery, and randomized to nonsurgical therapy—are then followed. One notable example of this design is the Spine Patient Outcomes Research Trial (SPORT) [33] addressing the comparative effectiveness of surgical and nonsurgical treatment for back pain attributable to herniated lumbar disk or spinal stenosis.

Ensuring that patients make informed decisions

As has been noted repeatedly, ensuring that the surgical decisions made by and with patients are fully informed is a challenge. Doctors and patients must work together, and to be successful despite real constraints of time and other obstacles, they need support in the form of knowledge management and decision aids. But there are skills and habits that surgeons can use to improve decision quality for their patients independent of the level of system support available for that purpose. Those habits and skills relate to the care with which the clinician works intentionally, first to minimize sources of unwarranted variation that tend degrade the extent to which decisions are knowledge-based and well informed, and second to recognize and accommodate sources of warranted variation that are essential to making decisions that are patient-centered and personalized. Other articles in this issue address approaches to reducing unwarranted variation—the design and conduct of relevant research, its management for timely availability to decision makers, and its accurate interpretation. This article has emphasized the importance of eliciting and honoring patients' personal valuations of alternative future health states, their attitudes to the specific risks and risk differences that are central to surgical decisions, and their attitudes to time trade-offs. The skills and habits necessary to accomplish this critical objective begin with nothing less than a genuine concern for patients, and an ability to relate to the unique meaning that the present illness and its treatment have in their lives.

References

[1] Mulley AG. Improving the quality of decision making. Journal of Clinical Outcomes Management 1995;2:9–10.
[2] Sepucha KR, Fowler FJ Jr, Mulley AG Jr. Policy support for patient-centered care: the need for measurable improvements in decision quality. Available at: http://www.healthaffairs.org. Accessed October 7, 2004.
[3] Braddock CH 3rd, Edwards KA, Hasenberg NM, et al. Informed decision making in outpatient practice: time to get back to basics. JAMA 1999;282(24):2313–20.

[4] McPherson K, Wennberg JE, Hovind OB, et al. Small-area variations in the use of common surgical procedures: an international comparison of New England, England, and Norway. N Engl J Med 1982;307(21):1310–4.

[5] Wennberg JE, Barnes BA, Zubkoff M. Professional uncertainty and the problem of supplier-induced demand. Soc Sci Med 1982;16:811–42.

[6] Mulley AG. Outcomes research: implications for policy and practice. In: Smith R, Delamothe T, editors. Outcomes into clinical practice. London: BMJ Publishing Group; 1995. p. 13–27.

[7] Fowler FJ, Wennberg JE, Timothy RP, et al. Symptom status and quality of life following prostatectomy. JAMA 1988;259:3018–22.

[8] Barry MJ, Mulley AG, Fowler FJ, et al. Watchful waiting versus immediate transurethral resection for symptomatic prostatism: the importance of patients' preferences. JAMA 1988;259:3010–7.

[9] Wennberg JE, Mulley AG, Hanley D, et al. An assessment of prostatectomy for benign urinary tract obstruction. Geographic variations and the evaluation of medical care outcomes. JAMA 1988;259:3018–22.

[10] Wasson JH, Reda DJ, Bruskewitz RC, et al. A comparison of transurethral surgery with watchful waiting for moderate symptoms of benign prostatic hyperplasia. The Veterans Affairs Cooperative Study Group on Transurethral Resection of the Prostate. N Engl J Med 1995;332(2):75–9.

[11] Barry MJ, Cockett ATK, Holtgrewe HL, et al. Relationship of symptoms of prostatism to commonly used physiologic and anatomic measures of benign prostatic hyperplasia. J Urol 1993;150:351–8.

[12] Barry MJ, Fowler FJ, O'Leary MP, et al. The American Urological Association symptom index for benign prostatic hyperplasia. J Urol 1992;148:1558–63.

[13] Barry MJ, Boyle P, Garraway M, et al. Epidemiology and natural history of BPH. In: Cockett ATK, Khoury S, Aso Y, et al, editors. The 2nd International Consultation on Benign Prostatic Hyperplasia (BPH). Jersey, Channel Islands (UK): Scientific Communication International Ltd; 1993. p. 17–34.

[14] Barry MJ. Benign prostatic hyperplasia: epidemiology and natural history. Urol Clin North Am 1990;17:495–507.

[15] Mulley AG. Assessing patients' utilities: can the ends justify the means? Med Care 1989;27: S269–81.

[16] O'Connor AM, Stacey D, Entwistle V, et al. Decision aids for people facing health treatment or screening decisions (Cochrane Review). In: The Cochrane Library, Issue 3. Oxford: Update Software; 2004.

[17] O'Connor AM, Stacey D, Entwistle V, et al. Decision aids for patients facing health treatment or screening decisions. Cochrane Database Syst Rev 2004;3:CD001431.

[18] O'Connor AM, Mulley AG Jr, Wennberg JE. Standard consultations are not enough to ensure decision quality regarding preference-sensitive options. J Natl Cancer Inst 2003;95:570–1.

[19] O'Connor A, Legare F, Stacey D. Risk communication in practice: the contribution of decision aids. BMJ 2003;327:736–40.

[20] Gigerenzer G, Edwards A. Simple tools for understanding risks: from innumeracy to insight. BMJ 2003;327:741–4.

[21] Schwartz L, Woloshin S, Welch G. Risk communication in clinical practice: putting cancer in context. J Natl Cancer Inst Monogr 1999;25:124–33.

[22] Steiner JF. Talking about treatment: the language of populations and the language of individuals. Ann Intern Med 1999;130:618–21.

[23] Edwards A, Elwyn G, Mulley A. Explaining risks: turning numerical data into meaningful pictures. BMJ 2002;324:827–30.

[24] Barry MJ, Cherkin DC, Chang Y, et al. A randomized trial of a multimedia shared decision-making program for men facing a treatment decision for benign prostatic hyperplasia. Dis Manag Clin Outcomes 1997;1:5–14.

[25] Barry MJ, Fowler FJ, Mulley AG, et al. Patient reactions to a program designed to facilitate patient participation in treatment decisions for benign prostatic hyperplasia. Med Care 1995; 33:771–82.

[26] Piercy GB, Deber R, Trachtenberg J, et al. Impact of a shared decision-making program on patients with benign prostatic hyperplasia. Urology 1999;53:913–20.

[27] Murray E, Davis H, See Tai S, et al. Randomised controlled trial of an interactive multimedia decision aid on benign prostatic hypertrophy in primary care. BMJ 2001;323:493–6.

[28] McNeil BJ, Weichselbaum R, Pauker SG. Speech and survival: tradeoffs between quality and quantity of life in laryngeal cancer. N Engl J Med 1981;305(17):982–7.

[29] Sepucha KR, Mulley AG. Extending decision support: preparation and implementation. Patient Educ Couns 2003;50(3):269–71.

[30] Fisher B, Redmond C, Poisson R, et al. Eight-year results of a randomized clinical trial comparing total mastectomy and lumpectomy with or without irradiation in the treatment of breast cancer. N Engl J Med 1989;320(13):822–8.

[31] Fisher B, Anderson S, Fisher ER, et al. Significance of ispilateral breast tumour recurrence after lumpectomy. Lancet 1991;338:327–31.

[32] Jacobson J, Danforth D, Cowan K, et al. Ten-year results of a comparison of conservation with mastectomy in the treatment of Stage I and II breast cancer. N Engl J Med 1995;332(14): 907–11.

[33] Birkmeyer NJO, Weinstein JN, Tosteson ANA, et al. Design of the Spine Patient Outcome Research Trial (SPORT). Spine 2002;27:1361–72.

SURGICAL
CLINICS OF
NORTH AMERICA

ELSEVIER
SAUNDERS

Surg Clin N Am 86 (2006) 193–199

Managing the Evidence Flood

Paul Glasziou, MD, PhD

Centre for Evidence-Based Practice, Department of Primary Health Care,
University of Oxford, Old Road Campus, Oxford OX3 7LF, England, UK

In their book *If Only We Knew What We Know*, O'Dell and Grayson [1] suggested four key reasons why knowledge is not transferred: (1) ignorance—we are not aware of existing useful knowledge, (2) lack of capacity—we do not have the resources or skills to implement the knowledge, (3) lack of relationship—lack of contact or trust in the sources of knowledge, and (4) lack of motivation—a perception that there is no need for change. All these reasons appear to be applicable in health care, though it is difficult to estimate their relative contribution [2]; however, because the first is a necessary preliminary step to overcome, this article focuses on it, to set it in the context of the others.

The problem of lack of transfer of knowledge is well-illustrated by the variations in surgical practice across areas and countries. For example, a recent survey of perioperative practices in five European countries [3] showed wide variation in practice, and that the majority of practice was at odds with current best evidence (in Fig. 1, evidence suggests the bars should approach 100%). Perioperative care is not unique in this respect, and such variations have been documented in virtually all specialties and in primary care.

If we have the same research base to work from, why do such variations in practice exist? There may be several reasons, but the critical first step is knowing about and accepting (or rejecting) the best research. If there were only a trickle of articles each year, then this would be straightforward—we could all read the same few articles and digest and debate these until a consensus was achieved. Unfortunately, in health care we are confronted not by a trickle but by a flood of new research. This flood can be measured by the number of new research articles that are published each year. Although we do not know the absolute global figures, we do know that each year there are now at least 560,000 new MEDLINE articles, including over 20,000 new randomized controlled trials. In daily terms, this means

E-mail address: paul.glasziou@dphpc.ox.ac.uk

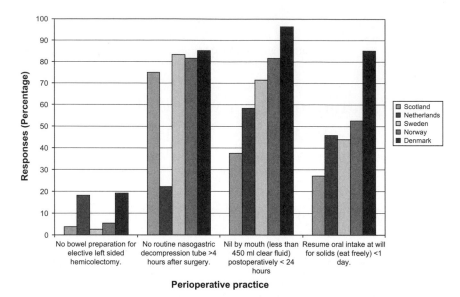

Perioperative practice

Fig. 1. Responses to questionnaire on perioperative care in colonic resections in five Northern European countries. Ideal would be 100% on each item. *From* Lassen K, Hannemann P, Ljungqvist O, et al, on behalf of the Enhanced Recovery After Surgery (ERAS) Group. Patterns in current perioperative practice: survey of colorectal surgeons in five northern European countries. BMJ 2005;330:1420; with permission.

about 1500 new MEDLINE articles, including 60 randomized trials, being published every day. Of course, not all of these are about surgery, but even searching Medline for articles in 2004 that include "surg" or "operat" in the title still leads to at least 89,886 surgical articles, or 246 per day. A search of the Cochrane library using the same terms suggests a cumulative total of at least 35,000 randomized trials related to surgery (out of a total of over 400,000 randomized trials). Hence there is no shortage of research to read, but there is a shortage of time to read it.

Of course not all this new research is about or relevant to surgery, but sorting out the articles that are relevant is not easy. It is not sufficient to read a few specialty journals, because much relevant research may be published in general medical journals, particularly the high-profile journals such as *The New England Journal of Medicine, The Journal of the American Medical Association, The BMJ (clinical research edition)*, and *Lancet*. The problem is illustrated by the journals involved in a recent systematic review of B-type natriuretic peptide as a diagnostic marker for heart failure [4]. The review identified 82 potential papers, 20 of which qualified but which were published in 16 different journals: five general medical journals (*The American Journal of Medicine, BMJ (clinical research edition), The Journal of the American Medical Association, Lancet, The New England Journal of Medicine*), nine cardiology journals (*The British Heart Journal, Circulation, Clinical Cardiology,*

The European Journal of Heart Failure, Hypertension, The Journal of Cardiac failure, The Journal of Hypertension, Revista Española de Cardiologia, Revisata Portuguesa de Cardiologia) and two noncardiology journals (*Age and Ageing, Clinica Chimica Acta*). Only 2 journals (*The British Medical Journal* and *Lancet*) had more than one of the articles. This is typical of the spread of publication across journals.

Managing the flood

So how can we manage the information overload and scatter? Information technologists suggest two possible modes of information management: "pull"—whereby we ask a specific question and seek out the answer, and "push"—whereby information is sent to us without a specific request. The evidence-based medicine (EBM) movement at McMaster University in Hamilton, Ontario, Canada largely focused on the former, that is the information pull. The standard textbooks of EBM [5] describe the four following steps:

Step 1. Convert the need for information (about prevention, diagnosis, prognosis, therapy, causation, etc) into an answerable question.

Step 2. Track down the best evidence with which to answer that question.

Step 3. Critically appraise that evidence for its validity (closeness to the truth), impact (size of the effect), and applicability (usefulness in our clinical practice)

Step 4. Integrate the critical appraisal with our clinical expertise and with our patient's unique biology, values and circumstances.

Often a fifth step is added, which is about monitoring how well we are doing at keeping track of and answering our own learning and information needs:

Step 5. Evaluate our effectiveness and efficiency in executing Steps 1–4, and seek ways to improve them both for next time.

These steps form the basic "pull" of evidence-based practice. We might also call this "just in time" learning; that is, finding the information we need only when we really need it. For example, if during case discussions the use of a new technique were mentioned, then you might assign someone on the surgical team to track down the evidence before the next case discussions. In this mode, evidence is only sought when it is relevant to the issues arising in practice. That is likely to be the most important and influential mode of learning, but we will also need some system to be kept abreast of important new research that introduces ideas we may never even ask questions about.

Box 1. Criteria for review and selection for abstracting

Prevention or treatment: quality improvement
Random allocation of participants to interventions
Outcome measures of known or probably clinical importance
  for 80% of the participants who entered the investigation

Diagnosis
Inclusion of a spectrum of participants, some, but not all,
  of whom have the disorder or derangement of interest
Each participant must receive the new test and the diagnostic
  standard test.
Either an objective diagnostic standard or a contemporary clinical
  diagnostic standard with demonstrably reproducible criteria
  for any subjectively interpreted component
Interpretation of the test without knowledge of the diagnostic
  standard result; interpretation of the diagnostic standard
  without knowledge of the test result

Prognosis
An inception cohort of persons, all initially free of the outcome
  of interest
Follow-up of 80% of patients until the occurrence of either
  a major study end point or the end of the study

Causation
Observations concerning the relation between exposures
  and putative clinical outcomes
Prospective data collection with clearly identified comparison
  groups for those at risk for the outcome of interest (in
  descending order of preference from randomized controlled
  trials, quasi-randomized controlled trials, nonrandomized
  controlled trails, cohort studies with case-by-case matching or
  statistical adjustment to create comparable groups, to nested
  case control studies
Masking of observers of outcomes to exposures (this criterion is
  assumed to be met if the outcome is objective)

Clinical prediction guides
The guide must be generated in one set of patients (training set)
  and validated in an independent set of real, not hypothetical,
  patients (test set).
The guide must pertain to treatment, diagnosis, prognosis, or
  causation.

Differential diagnosis
A cohort of patient who present with a similar, initially
  undiagnosed but reproducibly defined clinical problem
Clinical setting is explicitly described.
Ascertainment of diagnosis for 80% of patients using
  a reproducible diagnostic workup strategy and follow-up until
  patients are diagnosed, or follow-up of 1 month for acute
  disorders or 1 year for chronic or relapsing disorders

Systematic reviews
The clinical topic being reviewed must be clearly stated.
There must be a description of how the evidence on this topic
  was tracked down, from what sources, and with what inclusion
  and exclusion criteria.
One article included in the review must meet the above-noted
  criteria for treatment, diagnosis, prognosis, causation, quality
  improvement, or the economics of health care programs.

Filtering the flood

The complement to "pull" is the "push" of new information. But as indicated above, we need to be careful only to seek the small percentage of new research which is both valid and important. One way to glean the best from the flood of research information is to share the load. This principle has clearly been used in academic journal clubs across the world [6]; however, the most systematic research filtering process was developed by Brian Haynes at McMaster. After getting together colleagues to scan journals to find new articles that were both valid and relevant to clinical practice, he realized the end result was useful to other doctors. He approached the American College of Physicians and eventually persuaded them to produce an "evidence-based" supplement—*The ACP Journal Club*—that was provided free to all college members, and appeared six times yearly. The concept has since been adopted by several other groups, and we now also have *Evidence-Based Medicine* and *Evidence-Based Nursing* produced by the McMaster group, and several similar journals have arisen. It is worth looking in detail at the processes of one of these journals.

Today the filtering of the evidence-based journals has become an industrial-scale exercise. All the articles in over 120 journals are scanned. This list varies over time, as journals with low yield are dropped and new ones added. At least 50,000 new articles per year are scanned to check for the validity of the research methods. The article must pass the simple criteria shown in Box 1. For example, for research about treatment, the criteria ask for a randomized trial with at least 80% follow-up. Only around 2500 of the 50,000 articles pass the filtering criteria (that is about 5%), meaning a "noise reduction" filter of around 95%. This 1-in-20 pass rate means that most issues of most journals do not contain a single article that passes the validity criteria [7].

The second phase of filtering is to ask which of the 5% of articles that pass the basic validity criteria are also important. For this step, several active clinicians are asked to rate each article for: (1) its relevance to clinical practice; that is, whether and how much it might change practice; and (2) how newsworthy it is; that is, what proportion of colleagues are likely to already know this. For this relevance assessment, the articles are placed on a Web site, and then rated by several relevant specialists and generalists from the pool of nearly 4000 raters worldwide. If articles rate highly on both the relevance and newsworthiness scores, then they are picked for abstraction in the EBM journal. This involves rewriting the existing article as a structured abstract, and providing a commentary by a clinician expert in that topic.

Currently around 50% of therapy articles are about pharmaceutical treatment, and only around 5% are about surgery, but this reflects the generalist interests of the readers. Some examples of recent titles selected are

Surgery Was more Effective than Orthosis for Hallux Valgus

Stents Had Similar Clinical Outcomes but More Repeated Revascularisation than Did Bypass Surgery in Multivessel Disease

Surgery Was Associated with Greater Long Term Treatment Success than Wrist Splinting in Carpal Tunnel Syndrome

Prophylactic Coronary Artery Revascularisation Before Elective Vascular Surgery Did Not Improve Long Term Survival

Routine Testing Before Cataract Surgery Did Not Reduce Medical Adverse Events

Surgery Relieved Symptoms but Decreased Survival More than Medical Treatment in Gastro-oesophageal Reflux Disease

Review: Evidence Supports Surgery for Lumbar Disc Prolapse but Is Insufficient for Degenerative Lumbar Spondylosis

Review: Sparse High Quality Evidence Supports Surgery for Obesity

An evidence-based surgery journal?

Currently there is no journal of evidence-based surgery. So what should surgeons do while waiting for one? There are several possibilities. One is to join in the current McMaster Online Rating of Evidence (MORE) used for the EB journals mentioned above (hiru.mcmaster.ca/more/AboutMORE.htm), or to its downstream sister BMJ Updates (www.bmjupdates.com/). Both of these allow you to specify your clinical interest area, and provide means of alerting you to important new surgical articles relevant to your subspecialty.

You might want to go further, however, and replicate the process with colleagues for your own areas of interest. The author recommends using the filtering ideas of the EB journals to cut down on what you need to read, and then to share out the workload, so that each person is taking care of a single journal. That way, if you needed to look at the big five general medical journals, two or three general surgical journals, and two or three subspecialty journals, you would require a group of about 10 people to work together. If that is not possible at your hospital, you might consider joining forces with some other groups.

Whatever the means, our first problem is recognition that there is an inescapable and growing information problem. Unless we focus some of our research and practice effort on better organizing, filtering, and using the research we have the gap between what we know and what we do will continue to grow [2].

References

[1] O'Dell C, Grayson CJ. If only we knew what we know. New York: Free Press; 1998.
[2] Glasziou P, Haynes B. The paths from research to improved health outcomes. ACP J Club 2005;142(2):A8–10.
[3] Lassen K, Hannemann P, Ljungqvist O, et al, on behalf of the Enhanced Recovery After Surgery (ERAS) gtroup. Patterns in current perioperative practice: survey of colorectal surgeons in five northern European countries. BMJ 2005;330:1420–1.
[4] Doust JA, Glasziou PP, Pietrzak E, et al. A systematic review of the diagnostic accuracy of natriuretic peptides for heart failure. Arch Intern Med 2004;164(18):1978–84.
[5] Straus Se, Richardson WS, Glasziou PP, et al. Evidence based medicine: how to practice and teach EBM. 3rd edition. Edinburgh, Scotland: Churchill-Livingstone; 2005.
[6] Phillips RS, Glasziou P. What makes evidence-based journal clubs succeed? ACP J Club 2004; 140(3):A11–2.
[7] McKibbon KA, Wilczynski NL, Haynes RB. What do evidence-based secondary journals tell us about the publication of clinically important articles in primary healthcare journals? BMC Med 2004;2:33.

SURGICAL
CLINICS OF
NORTH AMERICA

Surg Clin N Am 86 (2006) 201–215

Surgical Decision-Making: Integrating Evidence, Inference, and Experience

John C. Marshall, MD

*Departments of Surgery and Critical Care Medicine, University of Toronto,
St. Michael's Hospital, 4th Floor Bond Wing, Room 4-007, 30 Bond Street, Toronto,
Ontario, Canada M5B 1W8*

Three surgeons were discussing a complication of a colleague: a leak following an emergency sigmoid resection and primary anastomosis for sigmoid diverticulitis with contained contamination. The patient was a 71-year-old man on antihypertensive therapy, known to have moderate chronic obstructive lung disease from a lifelong history of smoking, but otherwise active, and living independently with his spouse of close to 50 years.

"Clearly," said the first, "this was a serious lapse in judgment by Dr. X. I can't imagine what she must have been thinking when she decided to put the colon back together again. She put her patient at risk unnecessarily."

"I don't agree," said the second, "There is good evidence that anastomosis can be performed safely in unprepared bowel [1,2], even in the setting of diverticulitis and peritonitis [3]. This was a recognized complication, and simply reflects the fact that we will never eliminate complications entirely."

"Maybe," said the third, "but data from experimental studies show that fecal loading impairs anastomotic healing [4], especially in the setting of local inflammation [5]. The approach may be safe in ideal circumstances, but not in a man who has known comorbidities, and I would not have attempted an anastomosis here."

"The point is," snorted the first surgeon, "that in the real world, patients aren't experimental rats or even the carefully chosen subjects who are enrolled in clinical trials, but living, breathing humans who have plenty of associated health problems, who are operated on not by ultraspecialists in quaternary care centers, but by surgeons like me and you. You don't take chances; you do the safest thing possible, and for me, that would have been a Hartmann's procedure."

E-mail address: jc.marshall@uhn.on.ca

0039-6109/06/$ - see front matter © 2006 Elsevier Inc. All rights reserved.
doi:10.1016/j.suc.2005.10.009   *surgical.theclinics.com*

So—did the surgeon err in her judgment? What would have been the safest course of action? What would have been best for the patient? Is there a right answer, and how can we ever know?

This article explores the basis of surgical decision-making through the integration of evidence, inference, and experience—three complementary techniques for acquiring knowledge and applying it to a clinical problem. The elements of knowledge are complex, and also include intuition, and obedience—a menagerie of inputs whose acronym (EIEIO) brings to mind a children's song. Intuition is an indefinable capacity to predict the outcome of an event or decision, and derives from the integration of prior knowledge and experience, tempered by an innate capacity to establish the appropriate connections between disparate observations, and perhaps by some less tangible element of prescience. Obedience, on the other hand, is the uncritical adoption of the counsel of one's teachers and predecessors, typically expressed as aphorism or platitude: "Never let the sun set on a bowel obstruction"; "When in doubt, cut it out"; or "Big incisions for big surgeons." It may provide comfort for the neophyte, particularly when confronted with a difficult decision in an unusual case, but it rarely provides the insight that can help to inform a sophisticated therapeutic decision. For neither intuition nor obedience can be readily described, parsed, or taught, and both are beyond the scope of a discussion of the inputs that a surgeon has in making a clinical decision.

Evidence, inference, and experience are the methods through which observations are converted into the knowledge that informs decisions, and these three complementary approaches are our focus here.

Evidence, inference, and experience

Evidence, inference, and experience are not competing ideologies, but complementary methodologies for synthesizing empiric data (Fig. 1). Evidence is grounded in the principles of probability, whereas inference derives from those of logic; evidence is an example of inductive reasoning, and inference an example of deductive reasoning. Experience integrates these two principles, but its unique feature lies in the capacity to provide disproportionate weight to events that, although uncommon, are associated with substantial morbidity for the patient. Characteristics of evidence, inference, and experience are outlined in Box 1.

Inductive science and the methodologic basis of evidence-based medicine

Evidence-based medicine is defined as "the conscientious, explicit and judicious use of current best evidence in making decisions about the care of individual patients. The practice of evidence-based medicine means integrating individual clinical expertise with the best available external clinical evidence from systematic research" [6]. As a clinical tool, evidence-based

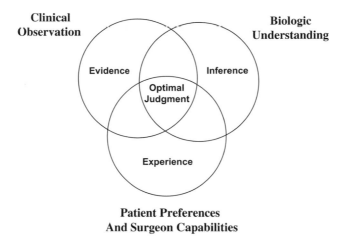

Fig. 1. Evidence, inference, and experience provide different, but complementary perspectives on the data that inform surgical decision-making: optimal decision-making occurs when the three are congruent.

medicine emphasizes the need to integrate the results of well-designed clinical trials with the capacity of the clinician to apply those findings to the unique circumstances of the individual patient—to integrate evidence with experience. Its particularly important contribution has been to codify the principles that underlie the generation of reliable clinical knowledge; these, in turn, derive from the application of the principles of probability and the scientific method to clinical research.

The methodologic basis of evidence-based medicine is inductive reasoning, and so the strongest evidence is that which arises from the most powerful tool of inductive science—the randomized controlled trial. Let us examine this more closely.

Inductive science is based on experimental observation and the application of principles of probability. Probability theory tells us that if one of two possible outcomes are equally likely—for example, the outcome of a coin toss being either heads or tails—then if the event is repeated numerous times, the number of each outcome should be approximately equal. If one were to flip a coin one hundred times, it would not be unexpected that the consequence might be 52 heads and 48 tails—this approximates the anticipated distribution of events if each is equally likely. But if the result were 80 heads and 20 tails, we would be suspicious that there was something amiss with the process—that the coin was loaded, or that the person tossing it was otherwise influencing the results. We can estimate the likelihood that deviations from the expected 50:50 ratio occur on the basis of random chance using a statistical test such as the χ^2 test. The probability of obtaining 52 heads as estimated by the χ^2 statistic is 0.89; or expressing it as an odds ratio, 1.08 (95% CI 0.62–1.89). On the other hand, the probability

---

Box 1. Evidence, inference, and experience

Evidence
Methods: frequentist
Focus: efficacy
Strengths: probabilistic, and therefore closest approximation to
    truth for group.
Weaknesses: probabilistic, and therefore may not represent best
    synthesis of information for an individual who does not meet
    specific characteristics of group, or who is an outlier in
    a population.

Inference
Methods: Bayesian
Focus: safety
Strengths: facilitates decision-making in absence of rigorous
    evidence. Permits refinement of evidence-based decisions.
Weaknesses: depends on assumptions of similarity; inherently
    subjective.

Experience
Methods: anecdotal
Focus: norms, and exceptions to the norm
Strengths: captures important, but as yet undefined elements of
    problem. Relates outcomes to individual surgeon's strengths
    and weaknesses.
Weaknesses: subservient to ego, hubris, and selective memory.

---

of obtaining 80 heads in 100 tosses is less than 0.0001 (odds ratio 4.00; 95% CI 2.14–7.49), or very unlikely indeed. Neither sequence of coin tosses can tell us with absolute certainty whether the process is being influenced by forces other than those of chance; it can only estimate the probability that the outcome observed reflects a purely random process.

Deviation from random chance forms the basis of scientific understanding. Indeed, biomedical research proceeds from the null hypothesis that there is no difference between two experimental groups, and draws inferences regarding mechanism or causality by rejecting the null hypothesis; in other words, by concluding that it is unlikely that observed differences occurred on the basis of chance alone. By convention, the level at which this cutoff is made (also known as the alpha level) occurs when the chance of differences representing random variability is less than one in twenty, or when the α level for probability (P) is less than 0.05. This value is purely arbitrary, representing a trade-off between increasing certainty and feasibility [7]. When the P value is 0.1, one can conclude that the probability that the observation occurred by chance is one in ten; conversely, when a study concludes that P is less than 0.05, this does not mean that the conclusion is true, but rather that there is less than a 5% chance, under the circumstances in which the study was performed, that the difference represented random chance. The distinction is subtle but important: there are no truths in medicine, merely assumptions whose probability is more or less secure.

The conclusion that an observed difference between two study populations reflects the consequences of an intervention can only be drawn with confidence when the populations are otherwise similar. Individuals within the study population will vary with regard to many characteristics—age, co-morbidities, gender, duration of illness, extent of disease, and genetic predisposition, along with many unmeasured factors—that may independently influence the outcome. The use of random allocation of patients to treatment groups provides the greatest likelihood that the resulting groups will be similar with respect to both known and unknown variables that might impact on the outcome of the intervention.

An evidence-based approach to the management of perforated diverticulitis

Let us apply an evidence-based approach to our patient who has perforated diverticulitis. Does the literature truly support the contention that primary anastomosis is as safe as the Hartmann's procedure?

A Medline search using the keywords "perforated diverticulitis, surgery," and restricting the search to studies in humans reported in the English literature, yields 152 citations. Many of these are case reports; one is a systematic review [3]. Because this latter is the most comprehensive, and likely to be the most rigorous, we will review it first.

Salem and Flum [3] reviewed 98 studies that provided comparisons of the Hartmann's procedure with resection and primary anastomosis for patients who had perforated peritonitis and significant peritoneal contamination (Hinchey stages 3 and 4). They noted substantial variability in the methodologic quality of the reports, and in the definitions and reporting of study outcomes. Nonetheless, when they pooled the results of studies for which data on survival and rates of infectious complications were available, they found that adverse outcomes were less frequent following primary anastomosis, particularly when the morbidity associated with colostomy reversal was considered (Table 1), and concluded that primary anastomosis is safe in selected patients who have perforated diverticulitis.

At first glance, it appears that the issue is settled: primary anastomosis has a mortality rate that is one half, and a wound infection that is one third that of the Hartmann procedure, albeit with a higher rate of anastomotic leakage—surely it should be the operative procedure of choice for our patient. Is it simple obstinacy, or the much vaunted surgical conservatism toward adopting changes in practice that drives our reluctance to embrace the practice unreservedly, or is there something more?

Table 1
Primary anastomosis versus the Hartmann procedure for perforated diverticulitis: a systematic review

Results	Hartmann	Hartmann + reversal	Primary anastomosis
Deaths	18.8%	19.6%	9.9%
Anastomotic leaks	—	4.3%	13.9%
Wound infection	24.2%	29.1%	9.6%

From Salem L, Flum DR. Primary anastomosis or Hartmann's procedure for patients with diverticular peritonitis? A systematic review. Dis Colon Rectum 2004;47(11):1953–64; with permission.

Discordance between the conclusions of systematic reviews [8], or of the conclusions of systematic reviews when compared with those of large, well-performed randomized controlled trials [9–11] is well-recognized. For example, systematic reviews of the efficacy of albumin supplementation in critical illness have variously concluded that supplementation is harmful [12], beneficial [13,14], or without obvious efficacy [15].

The divergent conclusions of these reviews can be attributed to multiple factors. These are outlined in Box 2.

Discordance can arise because of differences in the design and conduct of the studies that compose the systematic review. The intervention may vary from one study to the next—in the present review, for example, depending on whether a proximal diverting stoma was created in those patients who underwent primary anastomosis, whether an intraluminal stent was placed, and whether a colonic washout was performed.

The conclusions of a clinical trial are further influenced by the criteria used to select patients for entry into the study, the criteria used to exclude patients, and the outcome measures used to determine therapeutic efficacy. For example, the conclusions of a study comparing sigmoid resection and primary anastomosis with resection and colostomy for diverticular disease might be very different if the study population were all patients who had diverticular disease, or only patients who had perforated diverticulitis and established peritonitis. Even in the latter group, patients who had walled-off perforations might respond differently than patients who had diffuse purulent peritonitis. Exclusion criteria for a clinical trial—established to protect study subjects who might be at particularly high risk of adverse outcome— are typically quite variable from one study to the next, and so may disproportionately exclude those patients most likely to meet the study end points. Outcome measures are similarly variable, and even for such hard outcomes as death, conclusions may vary depending on whether mortality is measured early, at an intermediate time point such as 30 days or hospital discharge, or at a later date that might capture delayed events associated with colostomy closure.

Finally, and of particular relevance to the studies included in the present systematic review, studies in which treatment allocation is not established

---

Box 2. Sources of discordance in systematic reviews

Discordance arising from the original studies
Study design
    Intervention
    Target population
    Exclusion criteria
    Study definitions
    End points and outcome measures
    Randomization of study subjects
    Concealment of allocation
Study conduct
    Cointerventions
    Variability in clinical care
    Blinding of outcome adjudication
    Completeness of follow-up
Study reporting
    Completeness of report
    Publication bias

Discordance arising as a consequence of the systematic review
Studies selected
    Search strategy
    Inclusion of unpublished reports
    Exclusion criteria
Language of publications
Evaluation of quality
Selection of subgroups for analysis

---

randomly can yield misleading conclusions. None of the studies incorporated into the systematic review was a randomized controlled trial; it is entirely possible that selection bias occurred when patients were being considered for primary anastomosis or Hartmann's procedure, and that the higher-risk patients were more likely to undergo the latter intervention. Similarly, when historical controls are used, it is uncertain whether observed differences are attributable to the intervention, or to other unmeasured advances in the process of care.

The conclusions of a trial are also influenced by factors reflecting the conduct of the study, including blinding of outcome adjudication and the completeness of follow-up, as well as by regional differences in the process of care, or variability in cointerventions.

The conclusions of a systematic review are heavily dependent on the methods of the review itself. The study question may vary subtly between reviews, and the search strategies or criteria for including or excluding studies may differ. A decision to include or exclude unpublished studies, or to restrict the review to studies in the English language may also influence the conclusions. Further, the methods used to evaluate study quality, and to pool studies for subgroup analysis can influence the outcome of the review. Finally, pooling of aggregate data commonly requires a degree of subjective interpretation, and this too may impact on the inferences that are made.

So it would appear that the decision to perform a primary anastomosis was reasonable, based on the available evidence; however it is also apparent that, in the absence of solid data from adequately powered, randomized controlled trials, the evidentiary basis for making a decision in this particular case is weak, and dependent on inferences drawn from case series, and studies using historical controls.

Deductive science and inferential decision-making

Inferential approaches are probably the most commonly used methods for making surgical decisions in individual patients. Their need reflects the fact that for many of the most complex decisions that the surgeon must make, rigorous data from randomized controlled trials are simply unavailable, and when they are, the specific circumstances suggest the need to tailor the decision to the particular circumstances of an individual patient. Unlike evidence-based medicine, inference-based medicine lacks an articulated methodology; it may be presumptuous to suggest that such a methodology can be derived, but bear with me.

If the raw material that informs the practice of evidence-based medicine is inductive reasoning and the conclusions of randomized controlled trials, inference-based medicine depends on deductive reasoning and an understanding of the biology of health and disease [16]. These two approaches are complementary and interdependent. Inference provides a method for generating hypotheses that can be tested through randomized controlled trials, but it also provides a mechanism for making an informed decision in the absence of strong clinical evidence. Evidence-based approaches use the specific insights garnered from clinical trials and generalizes them to all similar patients. Inference-based approaches, on the other hand, integrate general principles derived from multiple data sources, and apply them to the specific problem at hand.

Inference-based thinking relies on principles of logic, but because it derives from biologic knowledge, is dependent on inductive, rather than deductive inference. Deductive inference provides conclusions that are necessarily true if the premises are true:

All men are mortal. Socrates is a man. Therefore Socrates is mortal

The truth of the first premise is accepted, as is that of the second, and therefore because the subject of the second—Socrates—is a subset of the first, the conclusion must be true.

With biologic inference, however, the reliability of the premises—drawn from experiment and observation—is less certain. The clinician creates an argument based on multiple premises that are believed to be accurate, and so reaches a conclusion that is likely to be true.

Our current question on the safety of primary anastomosis in perforated diverticulitis might be reformulated as a series of premises drawn from both experiment and clinical observation:

- Primary anastomosis can be performed safely in the unprepared bowel [2]; therefore fecal loading alone does not preclude primary anastomosis.
- Primary anastomosis can be performed safely in patients who have penetrating abdominal trauma [17,18]; therefore fecal spillage does not preclude anastomosis.
- Risk factors for anastomotic leakage include mechanical obstruction, chronic lung disease, alcohol abuse, transfusion, hypertension, ischemia, microvascular disease, and the use of drains [19–22].
- In experimental models, infection or inflammation have a modest inhibitory effect on wound healing [23,24].

We reach a conclusion similar to that which we had reached on the basis of a systematic review of clinical studies of the management of perforated diverticulitis—that primary anastomosis appears to be an acceptable option unless clinical factors such as mechanical obstruction, chronic lung disease, vascular disease, or large volume transfusion are prominent. None of the data we have used to reach this conclusion were derived from studies of patients who had diverticulitis; yet in aggregate, they create a convincing case that a decision to undertake a primary anastomosis is a reasonable one.

The focus of an inference-based approach to decision-making is patient safety, rather than therapeutic efficacy. Its primary use is in suggesting that a decision is unlikely to expose the patient to significant harm, rather than that it may improve clinical outcome. The randomized controlled clinical trial is the only reliable tool for determining the superiority of one treatment mode over another, because of the multiple potential sources of bias inherent in other experimental designs. With these principles in mind, we can formulate a series of questions to be considered in developing an inference-based approach to a particular problem. These are listed in Box 3.

Are there consistent mechanistic data from studies in animal models?

Animal models can provide insight into in vivo biology and its alteration by interventions that mimic disease; they do not replicate human disease, and they cannot reliably predict therapeutic efficacy [25]. Although specific biologic abnormalities can be reproduced in animals, disease is a complex process whose evolution reflects not only the biologic derangement, but also the genetic background and comorbidities of the host, and the response of the doctor in treating the clinical syndrome. The onset of perforated

---

Box 3. Inference-based analysis

Are there consistent mechanistic data from studies in animal models
- that characterize the biology of the process of interest?
- that evaluate the impact of physiologic perturbations or models of disease on the underlying biologic processes?

Are there human data to support the use of the approach of interest in a different disease process
- in a single disease with features of the problem to be addressed?
- or in a variety of disorders that reproduce discrete features of the problem?

What are the potential complications
- of the planned procedure?
- of the disease which is to be treated that might be made worse by the planned intervention?

What are the known risk factors for these complications
- from cohort and natural history studies?
- by analogy to other similar processes?

---

diverticulitis in humans, for example, may be gradual or abrupt, and the disease may be more or less advanced at the time of initial presentation. The extent of contamination is variable, as is the degree of host response to that contamination. The patient commonly has concomitant medical problems that may independently alter the host response. The patient is treated, with varying degrees of expertise, with intravenous fluids, antibiotics, and surgery or percutaneous drainage. Each of these factors modifies the clinical expression of the illness and therefore its potential to respond to specific therapy, and is extraordinarily difficult to replicate in an animal model.

Cecal ligation and puncture (CLP)—peritonitis induced by devascularization of the cecum by a ligature, and expression of feces by puncturing the ligated cecum with an 18 gauge needle—shares many features with perforated sigmoid diverticulitis [26]; however, its experimental rodent subjects are genetically similar, and undergo a single, standard insult. Experimental therapies are typically provided either before, or at a common time after the insult, and resuscitation, antibiotics, or surgical excision are often omitted. Indeed, animals that survive the initial insult begin to eat and gain weight by 4 days after the procedure, despite the presence of a gangrenous cecum within the peritoneal cavity. Thus inferences drawn from studies using CLP may provide insight into an in vivo response to a well-defined intervention, but the gulf between this insight and evidence of therapeutic relevance is wide.

Recognizing these important limitations, however, a preclinical model can provide important insights into how biologic processes evolve in vivo, and how defined perturbations affect that evolution. We can learn, for example, whether a colonic anastomosis will heal in the presence of peritonitis, and what specific elements of the healing process might be impacted.

Are there data supporting the use of the approach of interest in patients who have a different disease process?

The presence of underlying disease may modify the response to clinical intervention, but in general, evidence that an approach is safe in one group of patients will increase our confidence that it is safe in a different population. For example, the remarkable progress that has been made in the field of minimally invasive surgery over the past 2 decades reflects the fact that the safety and feasibility of laparoscopic abdominal surgery for cholecystectomy suggested that a similar approach could be safely applied to most intraperitoneal viscera.

Our confidence will be increased by evidence that the approach is safe in a variety of complementary clinical situations that reflect differing sources of potential risk to the patient. In our current discussion, for example, we wish to know not only that an intestinal anastomosis can be performed safely, but that the risk of leakage is acceptable despite potential risk factors such as fecal loading, emergency surgery, and active inflammation.

What are the potential complications of our plan of action?

Cohort studies and case series can provide valuable insight into the potential morbidity and mortality associated with a particular disease and its treatment. Understanding not only the short term risks and benefits, but also the longer-term impact on the patient's quality of life is important to planning an optimal approach.

The potential complications facing our patient who has perforated diverticulitis are many, but the one that drives the current debate is the risk of anastomotic leakage, and more precisely, the consequences of a leak, should it occur. We also consider risks such as that of wound infection or dehiscence or postoperative complications such as myocardial infarction or pulmonary embolism, and if percutaneous drainage of a localized perforation is technically feasible, we may infer that it is the optimal approach. It is important in the process of surgical decision-making to remember that the complications of the disease are not simply those faced at the initial operation, but also those resulting during subsequent procedures to restore intestinal continuity or to treat complications of our original management plan [27].

What are the known risk factors for these complications in other clinical settings?

Finally, inferential decision-making requires an appreciation of the factors that might increase the risk of adverse outcome in an individual patient. This information typically derives from cohort studies, and is strengthened by considering risk factors for adverse outcome from both the disorder of interest, and from related conditions in which similar therapies were applied.

Our evaluation of the risks of anastomotic failure revealed that patient factors such as hypertension, alcoholism, or vascular disease; clinical factors such as obstruction and ischemia; and therapeutic factors such as transfusion or the use of drains were all associated with an increased risk of anastomotic leakage. Importantly, inflammatory bowel disease or intraoperative spillage of gastrointestinal contents do not appear to increase the risk of anastomotic failure.

Experience: integrating subjectivity into surgical decision-making

Both evidence-based and inference-based approaches integrate insights derived from the structured and published work of other investigators; however, an individual surgeon's own experience figures centrally in the decisions that he or she makes, and influences the interpretation and application of surgical knowledge. Experience guides decision-making in three broad areas.

First, experience serves as an imperfect arbiter of published wisdom. It is this role that has created the greatest tension between the proponents and detractors of evidence-based medicine, for the counsel of experience is frequently at odds with the norms of evidence. Experience is shaped by consistency, but it is disproportionately influenced by the unanticipated and the exceptional. A surgeon will routinely perform a stapled colonic anastomosis because this is the technique she learned during her training, and because she has not experienced significant problems with the approach. But the occurrence of an anastomotic breakdown following a stapled low anterior resection will typically cause her to re-evaluate this approach, and perhaps even to perform a hand-sewn anastomosis or proximal diverting ileostomy for the next such patient. This decision does not reflect the acquisition of new knowledge that an alternate approach is superior, but rather the implicit assumption of a causal relationship between the decision (to undertake a stapled anastomosis) and the consequence (an anastomotic dehiscence). The important issue, however, is not whether there is a risk of dehiscence when a stapled anastomosis is performed, but whether that risk can be reduced with an alternate technique, a question that can only be reliably answered by a randomized controlled trial.

Second, experience serves to integrate published knowledge with the particular strengths, limitations, and values of the surgical practitioner. For example, although case series suggest that laparoscopic colectomy is as effective as an open procedure for patients who have diverticulitis [28,29], a surgeon may preferentially opt for one or other approach based on his or her level of comfort with the procedure.

Finally, experience provides a mechanism to tailor a therapeutic approach to the particular needs and values of the patient. Surgeons do not treat diseases; we treat patients who have diseases, and so the optimal approach will vary with the particular priorities of the patient. The decision to create a colostomy in an elderly patient whose dexterity is limited by arthritis, or whose eyesight is failing, may result in loss of independence or the need for institutionalization, and for some, this may be a fate worse than death.

Integrating evidence, inference, and experience

Evidence, inference, and experience provide complementary perspectives on the raw material that goes into a surgical decision, and the most secure decision is one for which all three support the choice that is made. The challenge arises when they do not.

Well-designed, adequately-powered, randomized controlled clinical trials provide the strongest evidence of therapeutic efficacy, but even where information from such trials is available, it is not necessarily definitive. Fully one sixth of influential randomized controlled trials published in the early 1990s have been contradicted by the results of subsequent investigation, whereas for a further one sixth, the magnitude of the effect has proven to be exaggerated [30]. Conversely, the absence of evidence from randomized controlled trials does not invalidate an otherwise supportable conclusion: the absence of such evidence for parachutes is unlikely to convince even the most ardent enthusiast of evidence-based medicine to jump from a plane without one [31]! Because of the assumptions inherent in their design, randomized trials are best suited to answering questions applicable to populations, rather than to individual patients. Thus they provide particularly strong support for interventions that are prophylactic in nature, or therapeutic in more homogeneous patient populations, and must be interpreted more carefully when the results are used to make treatment decisions in the individual patient [32].

The results of clinical trials are but one piece of a body of information that supports a particular conclusion, and must be interpreted within that totality. Indeed this concept is inherent in the Bayesian approach to statistical inference, in which the strength of the conclusions are evaluated in the context of the prior probability of the truth of the experimental hypothesis using a Bayes factor or likelihood ratio [33]. For a single data set such as the results of a trial, Bayesian analysis affords greater confidence in the conclusions when these are consistent with what is known than when they are divergent, thus marrying evidence and inference, and mirroring the well-recognized conservatism of clinicians in adopting new approaches based on trial results that are at odds with what is expected. On the other hand, prior understanding—whether based on inference or experience—may be flawed, selective, and unduly influenced by obedience to preconceptions, and so uncertainty and controversy is an inescapable element in the evaluation of medical information.

The integration of evidence, inference, and experience does not provide the truth, or even point to a preferred approach to the management of an individual patient—what it does is to shift the fulcrum around which clinical decisions are made. Our review of the experimental and clinical literature on primary anastomosis for perforated diverticulitis does not tell us what we should do in this case, and in particular, provides no guarantee that one option will avoid complications. But it does tell us that the option is reasonable, and frees us to make the decision that will provide the best solution for this particular patient.

References

[1] Zmora O, Mahajna A, Bar-Zakai B, et al. Colon and rectal surgery without mechanical bowel preparation: a randomized prospective trial. Ann Surg 2003;237(3):363–7.

[2] Bucher P, Mermillod B, Gervaz P, et al. Mechanical bowel preparation for elective colorectal surgery: a meta-analysis. Arch Surg 2004;139(12):1359–64.

[3] Salem L, Flum DR. Primary anastomosis or Hartmann's procedure for patients with diverticular peritonitis? A systematic review. Dis Colon Rectum 2004;47(11):1953–64.

[4] Ravo B, Metwall N, Yeh J, et al. Effect of fecal loading with/without peritonitis on the healing of a colonic anastomosis: an experimental study. Eur Surg Res 1991;23(2):100–7.

[5] Feres O, Monteiro dos Santos JC Jr, Andrade JI. The role of mechanical bowel preparation for colonic resection and anastomosis: an experimental study. Int J Colorectal Dis 2001; 16(6):353–6.

[6] Sackett DL, Rosenberg WM, Gray JA, et al. Evidence based medicine: what it is and what it isn't. BMJ 1996;312(7023):71–2.

[7] Goodman SN. Toward evidence-based medical statistics. 1: The P value fallacy. Ann Intern Med 1999;130(12):995–1004.

[8] Jadad AR, Cook DJ, Browman GP. A guide to interpreting discordant systematic reviews. CMAJ 1997;156(10):1411–6.

[9] Cook DJ, Reeve BK, Guyatt GH, et al. Stress ulcer prophylaxis in critically ill patients. Resolving discordant meta-analyses. JAMA 1996;275(4):308–14.

[10] Cook DJ, Guyatt GH, Marshall JC, et al. A randomized trial of sucralfate versus ranitidine for stress ulcer prophylaxis in critically ill patients. N Engl J Med 1998;338:791–7.

[11] Lelorier J, Gregoire G, Benhaddad A, et al. Discrepancies between meta-analyses and subsequent large randomized, controlled trials. N Engl J Med 1997;337(8):536–42.

[12] Schierhout G, Roberts I. Fluid resuscitation with colloid or crystalloid solutions in critically ill patients: a systematic review of randomised trials. BMJ 1998;316:961–4.

[13] Haynes GR, Navickis RJ, Wilkes MM. Albumin administration—what is the evidence of clinical benefit? A systematic review of randomized controlled trials. Eur J Anaesthesiol 2003;20(10):771–93.

[14] Vincent JL, Navickis RJ, Wilkes MM. Morbidity in hospitalized patients receiving human albumin: a meta-analysis of randomized, controlled trials. Crit Care Med 2004;32(10): 2029–38.

[15] Alderson P, Bunn F, Lefebvre C, et al. Human albumin solution for resuscitation and volume expansion in critically ill patients. Cochrane Database Syst Rev 2004 Oct 18;(4):CD001208.

[16] Marshall JC, Girotti MJ. From premise to principle: the impact of the gut hypothesis on the practice of critical care surgery. Can J Surg 1995;38:132–41.
[17] Demetriades D, Murray JA, Chan L, et al. Penetrating colon injuries requiring resection: diversion or primary anastomosis? An AAST prospective multicenter study. J Trauma 2001; 50(5):765–75.
[18] Maxwell RA, Fabian TC. Current management of colon trauma. World J Surg 2003;27(6): 632–9.
[19] Gooszen AW, Tollenaar RA, Geelkerken RH, et al. Prospective study of primary anastomosis following sigmoid resection for suspected acute complicated diverticular disease. Br J Surg 2001;88(5):693–7.
[20] Sorenson LT, Jorgensen T, Kirkeby LT, et al. Smoking and alcohol abuse are major risk factors for anastomotic leakage in colorectal surgery. Br J Surg 1999;86(7):927–31.
[21] Golub R, Golub RW, Cantu R Jr, et al. A multivariate analysis of factors contributing to leakage of intestinal anastomoses. J Am Coll Surg 1997;184(4):364–72.
[22] Fawcett A, Shembekar M, Church JS, et al. Smoking, hypertension, and colonic anastomotic healing; a combined clinical and histopathological study. Gut 1996;38(5):714–8.
[23] Hesp FL, Hendriks T, Lubbers EJ, et al. Wound healing in the intestinal wall. Effects of infection on experimental ileal and colonic anastomoses. Dis Colon Rectum 1984;27(7):462–7.
[24] Witte MB, Barbul A. Repair of full-thickness bowel injury. Crit Care Med 2003;31(Suppl 8): S538–46.
[25] Marshall JC. Modeling MODS: what can be learned from animal models of the multiple-organ dysfunction syndrome? Intensive Care Med 2005;31(5):605–8.
[26] Wichterman KA, Baue AE, Chaudry IH. Sepsis and shock—a review of laboratory models and a proposal. J Surg Res 1980;29:189–201.
[27] Shellito PC. Complications of abdominal stoma surgery. Dis Colon Rectum 1998;41(12): 1562–72.
[28] Pugliese R, Di Lernia S, Sansonna F, et al. Laparoscopic treatment of sigmoid diverticulitis: a retrospective review of 103 cases. Surg Endosc 2004;18(9):1344–8.
[29] Scheidbach H, Schneider C, Rose J, et al. Laparoscopic approach to treatment of sigmoid diverticulitis: changes in the spectrum of indications and results of a prospective, multicenter study on 1545 patients. Dis Colon Rectum 2005;47(11):1883–8.
[30] Ioannidis JPA. Contradicted and initially stronger effects in highly cited clinical research. JAMA 2005;294(2):218–28.
[31] Smith GC, Pell JP. Parachute use to prevent death and major trauma related to gravitational challenge: systematic review of randomised controlled trials. BMJ 2003;327(7429):1459–61.
[32] Dans AL, Dans LF, Guyatt GH, et al. Users' guides to the medical literature: XIV. How to decide on the applicability of clinical trial results to your patient. JAMA 1998;279(7):545–9.
[33] Goodman SN. Toward evidence-based medical statistics. 2: The Bayes factor. Ann Intern Med 1999;130(12):1005–13.

ELSEVIER
SAUNDERS

Surg Clin N Am 86 (2006) 217–220

SURGICAL
CLINICS OF
NORTH AMERICA

Epilogue

Evidence-Based Surgical Practice and Patient-Centered Care: Inevitable

Sir Muir Gray, CBE, DSc, MD, FRCP,
FRCPS(Glasgow)
Jonathan L. Meakins, OC, MD, DSc, FRCS(Hon),
FRCS(C,Glasgow)

The authors started by asking if evidence-based surgery was inevitable. We believe it is, and have created a basic fishtail diagram (Fig. 1) over which the articles of this issue of *Surgical Clinics of North America* have fleshed out a framework for the delivery of good-quality health care.

By the 1990s, systems development had evolved significantly (Fig. 2). Pressures were exerted by funding agencies, either federal or private insurance, to refine systems and processes of care. Patient safety, defining standards, and a recognition that change was in the air were supported by professional development. This evolution by clinicians was substantially influenced by public pressure and increasing lay involvement in professional bodies and regulating agencies. Slowly the view of outcomes became less doctor-centered.

Concurrently, a more focused approach to the application of knowledge (Fig. 3) became apparent. The significance of the evidence-based medicine or surgery movement started to be recognized. Protocols, clinical guidelines, or care maps could no longer be defined by the views of an idiosyncratic individual. Others on the service would balk; nurses and allied health professionals might even demand evidence. To support changing clinical pathways, there had to be evidence (knowledge from research) blended with data and experience.

The patient safety movement is similarly supported by knowledge from data—statistics on the incidence of error in patient management. Hospitals are extraordinarily complex organizations. The creation of the systems to reduce error requires the application of knowledge, not only to deliver best practice, but also to reduce untoward events in the midst of complexity.

The ultimate image is the evolution to patient-centered outcomes (Fig. 4). With communication of the many options that exist for most clinical

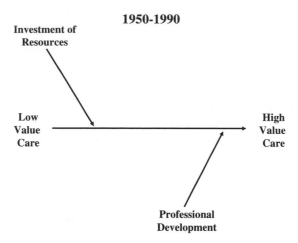

Fig. 1. Health care delivery diagram.

entities, the informed patient will be an integral part of decision-making. This will drive the measurement of outcomes to be increasingly patient-centered. A good example of surgeon-centered versus patient-centered outcome is seen in hernia repairs. The surgeon's measure is recurrence, but for the patient it could well be complete absence of pain (symptoms). Specifically, tension-based (Shouldice, Bassini, Cooper's) ligament repairs can have low recurrence rates, but a significant incidence of chronic discomfort or pain. In cancer care, some patients will trade longevity for quality of life, or will want to exchange the risk of one class of complications for another.

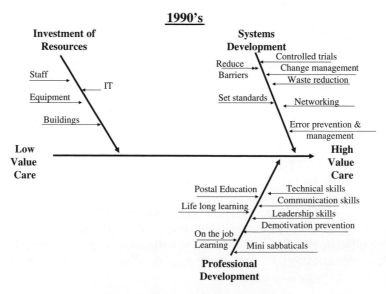

Fig. 2. Systems development diagram.

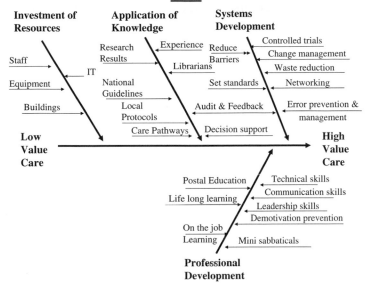

Fig. 3. Application of knowledge diagram.

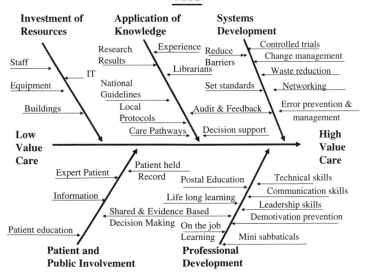

Fig. 4. Patient-centered outcomes diagram.

Shared decision-making is integral to future surgical care. It is not possible without the organization and applications of knowledge. Evidence-based surgical practice is inevitable as practice and outcomes become patient-centered.

Sir Muir Gray, CBE, DSc, MD, FRCP, FRCPS(Glasgow)
Jonathan L. Meakins, OC, MD, DSc, FRCS(Hon), FRCS(C,Glasgow)
Nuffield Department of Surgery, University of Oxford
Oxford, England, UK

E-mail addresses: muir.gray@dphpc.ox.ac.uk (M. Gray);
jonathan.meakins@nds.ox.ac.uk (J.L. Meakins)

ELSEVIER
SAUNDERS

SURGICAL
CLINICS OF
NORTH AMERICA

Surg Clin N Am 86 (2006) 221–225

Index

Note: Page numbers of article titles are in **boldface** type.